SURVIVAL GUIDE TO
ACUTE MEDICINE

SURVIVAL GUIDE TO ACUTE MEDICINE

Edited by

Lee Kang Hoe, John Wong, Tan Chorh Chuan

*Departments of Medicine & Medical Oncology,
National University Hospital, Singapore*

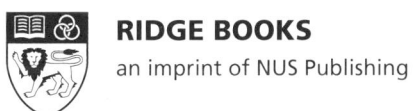

RIDGE BOOKS
an imprint of NUS Publishing

© Singapore University Press
  an imprint of NUS Publishing
  National University of Singapore
  AS3-01-02, 3 Arts Link
  Singapore 117569

  Fax: (65) 6774-0652
  E-mail: nusbooks@nus.edu.sg
  Website: http://www.nus.edu.sg/npu

  First Edition 1998
  First Reprint 1999
  Second Reprint 2002
  Third Reprint 2003
  Fourth Reprint 2004
  Fifth Reprint 2006

ISBN 9971-69-220-1 (Paper)

Typeset by : Scientifik Graphics
Printed by : Photoplates Pte Ltd

Dedication

To our ever patient wives and families

CONTENTS

Pulmonary

Renal

Neurology

Gastrointestinal

FOREWORD

The care of acutely ill patients constitutes a substantial part of the "on-duty" housestaff and "on-call" specialists. In these patients, their condition may evolve rapidly with the development of life-threatening crisis. A rapid reference guide in such circumstances therefore becomes necessary, both for the patient's, as well as for the doctor's "survival".

Acute medical problems essentially fall under two categories: diagnostic or therapeutic. After the immediate question, "Are the vital signs stable?" you might want to elucidate the following questions: "What is the cause of the chest pain? Why is the blood pressure low? How should we manage the case? What investigations should be ordered? Which drugs to give? When to give?" In instances with a known disease, "What complications have arisen? How to investigate and treat this disease." You will find a ready and succinct answer to most of the common emergent medical conditions in this book.

This volume is authored by practising physicians, each with many years of experience dealing with such emergent, general, as well as multi-specialty, problems. The format is a practical one with a problem-solving approach.

I sincerely hope you will find this handy volume useful the next time you go "on-duty" or are called upon to assess an acutely ill patient. You will no doubt "survive" if not "thrive" in these future encounters. I am confident that this edition will be the first of several in the years to come.

Professor Chan Heng Leong
1998

LIST OF ABBREVIATIONS

abdo — change to abdomen

bd
bid po } twice a day

dl — decilitre

Hb — Haemoglobin
Hct — Haematocrit

IV — intravenous/intravenously

prn — as required
pts
ptx } patients

qds
qid po } four times a day
q8hrs — 8 hourly

stat — immediately

tds/tid — three times a day

A-V — arteviovenous
ABG — Arterial blood gas
ACE — angiotensin converting enzyme
ACLS — advanced cardiac life support
ACTH — adrenocorticotrophic hormone
ADR — adverse drug reaction
AFB — acid fast bacillus
AHA — American Heart Association
ALF — acute liver failure
AMI — acute myocardial infarction

ANA — anti-nuclear antibody
ANCA — antineutrophil cytoplasmic auto antibody
AXR — abdominal X-ray

BBB — Blood brain barrier
BCLS — Basic Cardiac LifeSupport
BID — bid
BP — blood pressure

CI — cardiac index
CHF — congestive heart failure
CK — creatinine kinase
CKMB — creatinine kinase (MB)
CNS — central nervous system
COPD — chronic obstructive pulmonary disease
CPAP — continuous positive airway pressure
CXR — chest X-ray
CVP — Central venous pressure
CT — computer tomography

DDAVP
DIC/DIVC — Disseminated intravascular coagulation
DKA — Diabetic ketoacidosis

ECG — electrocardiogram
ESRF — End stage renal failure
ETEC — enterotoxigenic E coli

FBC — Full blood count
FEV_1 — Forced expiratory volume in 1sec.

GI — gastrointestinal
GTN — glyceryyl trinitrate

HBV — Hepatitis B virus
HHH — high high high
HHNK — hyperosmolar hyperglycaemic Non ketotic
HIV — human immunodoficiency virus
HR — heart rate

IABP — intra-aortic balloon pump
ICH — intracranial hemorrhage
ICP — intracranial pressure
ICU — intensive care unit
IU — International Units

JVP — jugular venous pressure

LA — left atrium
LAM — lymphagiomyomatosis
LBBB — left bundle branch block
LDH — lactate dehydrogenase
LFT — Liver function test
LPFB — Left posterior fascicular block
LV — left ventricle
LVH — left ventricular hypertrophy

MAP — mean airway pressure
MCTD — mixed connective tissue disease
MICU — medical intensive care unit
MR — mitral regurgitation
MRI — Magnetic Resonance Imaging

NPPV — Noninvasive positive pressure ventilation
NSAID — Nonsteroidal anti-inflammatory drug

OGD — oesophagogastroduodenoscopy

PA — Pulmonary artery
tPA — tissue plasminogen activator
PAM — Pralidoxime
PAP — Peak airway pressure
PAWP — Pulmonary artery wedge pressure
PCP — Pneumocystiis carinii pneumonia
PD — Peritoneal dialysis
PE — Pulmonary embolism
PEA — Pulseless electrical activity
PEEP — Positive end-expiratory pressure

PEFR — Peak expiratory flow rate
Phx — Past Medical history
PMN — Polymorphonuclear neutrophil
PPF — Plasma protein fraction
PTC — Percutaneous transhepatic cholangiogram
PTCA — Percutaneous transluminal coronary angioplasty
PT/PTT/aPTT — Prothrombin time
PR — per rectum

Q wave
q wave

RA — right atrium
RBBB — right bundle branch block
RBC — red blood cell
ROSC — return of spontaneous circulation

SAH — subarachnoid hemorrhage
SBP — systolic blood pressure
SIADH — Syndrome of inappropriate anti-diuretic hormone
SIRS — Systemic inflammatory response syndrome
SK — streptokinase
SLE — systemic lupus erythematosis
SVC — superior vena cava

TB — tuberculosis

U/S — ultra-sound
UTI — urinary tract infection

VF ventricular fibrillation
VQ — ventilation — perfusion
VSD — ventricular septal defect
VT — Ventricular tachycardia

WBC — white blood cell
WG — Wegener's granulomatosis
WWF — Weil — Widal Felix

APPROACHES AND EVALUATION

ACUTE CHEST PAIN
LEE KANG HOE

Attempt to make a diagnosis and exclude the severe causes.

Clinical evaluation
1. Look at the patient and decide whether they look ill.
2. Check the vitals signs, while taking a quick history.
3. History: try to establish the site, nature, precipitating factor, length for the pain; ask for previous history; try to localise the origin for the pain — cardiac, lungs, pleural, oesophagus, abdominal, chest wall (skin, muscles, bones).
4. Direct your examination accordingly. Look for pericardial or pleural rub; pneumothorax, dissecting aneurysm, acute abdomen, rib fractures, etc.

Investigations
1. FBC, CK and CKMB, electrolytes, urea and creatinine.
2. ECG — ST elevation or depression.
3. Chest X-ray.

Management
1. IV plug.
2. Oxygen if patient unwell.
3. Make a diagnosis and treat underlying cause, e.g. GTN sublingual for angina. Most important to exclude AMI, aortic dissection, and pulmonary embolism.
4. Recheck patient for resolution of symptom and not worsening.
5. Have a high suspicion for ischemic heart disease.

ACUTE BREATHLESSNESS AND ACUTE RESPIRATORY FAILURE
LIM TOW KEANG

Dyspnoea
Subjective feeling of discomfort associated with breathing, as distinct from tachypnoea and hyperventilation.

Clinical evaluation
1. Exclude upper airway obstruction. Secure patency of upper airway.
2. Check BP, pulse rate and for pallor and signs of shock (remember that anaemia, sepsis and pre-shock can cause dyspnoea). Take measures to keep patient haemo-dynamically stable.
3. Establish if patient has: dyspnoea of acute onset — asthma, pneumothorax, heart failure, pulmonary embo-lism, metabolic acidosis OR; chronic effort-related dyspnoea exacerbated by minimal effort — underlying COLD or poor cardiac reserve presenting suddenly with dyspnoea brought on by a rare stint of exercise or an inter-current illness, e.g. sepsis.

Investigations
1. Blood: FBC, electrolytes, urea and creatinine, ABG (pulse oximetry), cardiac enzymes (if indicated).
2. Imaging: CXR.
3. ECG.

Acute respiratory failure
HYPOXEMIA: $PaO_2 < 60$ mm Hg and/or arterial O_2 saturation $< 92\%$.
HYPERCAPNIA: $PaCO_2 > 50$ mm Hg; severe if pH also < 7.30 also
Type I: Hypoxemia without hypercapnia
Type II: Hypercapnia with hypoxemia.

Management

1. Administer oxygen with target PaO_2 > 65 mmHg and/or arterial O_2 saturation 92%–95% (see Oxygen therapy). For severe hypoxemia alone, start with high FiO_2 and titrate according to pulse oximeter or arterial blood gas results. Artificial ventilation should be considered if hypoxemia not correctable with oxygen therapy.
2. For hypercapnic respiratory failure, give oxygen cautiously with frequent monitoring of arterial blood gases because of the danger of worsening CO_2 retention and narcosis.
3. Artificial ventilation (invasive and noninvasive methods) MUST be considered in: patients who present with mental obtundation and frank respiratory narcosis, and patients who deteriorate (more confused, rising $PaCO_2$, pH falling to < 7.25) during treatment or O_2 therapy. O_2 therapy should be reduced but NOT stopped abruptly.
4. Identify and treat cause(s) of acute respiratory failure.
5. Common causes of hypoxemia are: pneumonia, pulmonary oedema, pulmonary embolism, poor cardiac output, airway obstruction.
6. Common causes of hypercapnic respiratory failure are: V/Q mismatch — COLD, cardiogenic pulmonary oedema; hypoventilation — narcotic drug overdose; neuromuscular weakness, e.g. myasthenia, Gullain-Barre syndrome; mixed mechanisms — e.g. sedation in COLD patient.

Oxygen therapy

Device	Advantages	Disadvantages	Common Indications
Nasal prongs	Simple to use Free access to mouth Compliance better	Imprecise FiO_2 Maximum FiO_2 < 40%	Less hypoxic patients Patients with V/Q mismatch (e.g. COLD) or hypoventilation (e.g. narcotic toxicity)
Venturi nasal mask	More precise FiO_2 Maximum FiO_2 50%	Needs 2 settings* Poorer compliance	Controlled oxygen therapy e.g. with hypercapnic respiratory failure from COLD

Device	Advantages	Disadvantages	Common Indications
Rebreathing mask	FiO_2 up to 80%		
Mask-CPAP system	FiO_2 up to 40–100% + CPAP 5–10 cm H_2O		Severe hypoxia from intrapulmonary shunts (e.g. ARDS, pulmonary oedema)

* Correct application for venturi masks:

1. Decide on the FiO_2 desired (24% to 30% — use green diluter on mask; 35% to 50% use white diluter).
2. Set oxygen to appropriate flow-rate for FiO_2 desired.
3. Set the size of the venturi aperture on the face mask to the desired FiO_2.

ACUTE ABDOMINAL PAIN
LIM SENG GEE

Introduction
The pain may originate from causes within the abdomen and outside the abdomen. Many conditions may lead to abdominal pain. The main differential is to exclude a surgical abdomen that requires laparotomy.

Clinical evaluation
1. History: determine whether first episode or acute presentation of chronic pain (> 3 months duration); identify characteristics and localisation of pain; relationship to bowels and and food intake; previous operations.
2. Physical: establish the location, look for masses, previous surgery, do a rectal examination, exclude a surgical abdomen (tender, guarding with peritonism (rebound), absent bowel sounds, compatible history).
3. Look for fever, anemia, haematemesis ± malaena, jaundice, weight loss, hematuria.
4. Common causes to remember: peptic ulcer disease (epigastric, usually "hunger pains" or indigestion, associated with food, nocturnal pain, periodicity, relief by milk, alkali or food, only 30%–50% of patients have classical or typical symptoms), acute cholecystitis/biliary colic, pylonephritis/renal colic, pancreatitis, gastroenteritis, non-ulcer dsypepsia [meal-related, associated bloating and gas, intolerance to specific foods — spicy foods, coffee, fatty foods, acid drinks, usually long history (months to years), absence of weight loss and fever], irritable bowel syndrome [at least 3 months, abdominal pain relieved by defecation, ±change in stool frequency, ± change in stool consistency plus at least 2 of the following — altered stool frequency, altered stool form (soft -watery), altered stool passage (straining, urgency, incomplete evacuation), mucous, bloating or distention], musculoskeletal pain/fibromyalgia (worse with movement,

exercise and coughing, localised/focal muscular tenderness).

5. Non-abdominal causes: cardiac (CAD, pericarditis), torsion of testes, pneumonia, diabetic ketoacidosis, porphyria, uraemia.

Investigations

1. Laboratory investigations: FBC, liver function test, electrolytes, urea and creatinine, amylases. PT, PTT and X-match if bleed likely or surgical abdomen.
2. Appropriate cultures — blood, stool, urine.
3. Imaging: AXR, (erect CXR for free air if perforation suspected), U/S or CT scan as dictated by diagnosis.
4. Others: OGD, barium study, manometry as indicated.

Management

1. Treat the underlying cause.

peptic ulcer	H_2 blocker, antacids, H.pylori eradication
cholecystitis	refer for surgery
pancreatitis	nil by mouth, iv fluids, iv somatostatin (see chapter)
pylonephritis	iv antibiotics
renal colic	iv pethidine, iv buscopan
gastroenteritis	observation, may treat with loperamide 2mg prn.
Non-ulcer dyspepsia	cisapride, domperidone, antacids, H_2 blockers
Irritable bowel syndrome	mebeverine, benzodiazepine
fibromyalgia	NSAIDs, tricyclic anti-depressants
non-specific abdominal pain	antacids, H_2 blockers

2. Surgical abdomen requires a laparotomy.
3. Resuscitate if hemodynamically unstable.

CONFUSION AND COMA
RICHARD CHAN and HO KING HEE

Definition
1. Confusion refers to a mental state characterised by disorientation to either time, place or person, that is not explained by normal forgetfulness or inattention.
2. Delirium is an exacerbated state of confusion, associated with incoherent thought, hallucination and/or autonomic instability.
3. Coma is a state of total unresponsiveness to verbal, tactile and noxious stimuli.

Differential diagnosis
Confusional state should be differentiated from delusion, hallucination and receptive aphasia.

Exclude lock-in state (bilateral basis pontine lesion) before declaring a patient to be comatose.

Clinical evaluation
1. General examination to look for evidence of sepsis (abdomen, chest), drug abuse (smell, needle tracks), trauma (hematoma, laceration).
2. Neurological examination to look for focal deficit — pay particular attentions to pupillary reflexes, eye movement, corneal reflexes, lateralised weakness, plantar responses. Coma and confusion can be caused by similar disease processes. In the absence of a metabolic/toxicologic cause, coma is likely due to a structural lesion affecting the reticular formation in the brain stem, or involving most cortical surface in both cerebral hemispheres. Common or important causes of confusion and coma are:
   (i)   Sepsis.   Important to rule out intra-abdominal sepsis or pneumonia, particularly in the elderly.
   (ii) Metabolic disturbances.   Hypoglycaemia, hyponatraemia, hypernatraemia, hypocalcemia, hyper-

calcaemia, hepatic encephalopathy, hypothyroidism, hyperthyroidism ("thyroid storm").

(iii) Global cerebral hypoxia/hypoperfusion. Acute hypoxia from any cause (acute respiratory failure), hypotension, systemic embolisation (e.g. fat/air embolism), severe anaemia.

(iv) Drug Overdose/Withdrawal. Remember ethanol, methanol, CNS stimulant (amphetamines, cocaine), sedatives (benzodiazepine, antihistamines), anti-depressant (tricyclic amines), anticonvulsants, antipsychotics, etc.

(v) Cerebral trauma. Concussion, cerebral contusion, subdural/epidural hemorrhage.

(vi) CNS infection. i.e. meningitis, encephalitis, brain abscess.

(vii) Seizure disorder/post ictal state. Particularly if the focus lies in the mesial temporal cortex.

(viii) Stroke. Including cerebral infarct, intracerebral hemorrhage and subarachnoid hemorrhage.

Investigation

1. Blood glucose (hypocount), FBC, electrolytes, urea and creatinine, calcium, LFT, ABG, toxicology screen (including alcohol), blood culture, ammonia level.
2. Urine for culture, toxicology screen.
3. ECG to rule out acute myocardial infarction.
4. Chest X-ray to rule out pneumonia.
5. CT head scan to rule out structural lesion (tumor, stroke, hemorrhage), look for mass effect/midline shift.
6. Lumbar puncture to rule out CNS infection.

Management

1. Ensure adequacy of airway support and circulation.
2. IV access ± IV fluids (depends on hydration status).
3. Keep nil by mouth.
4. Management is mainly supportive. Definitive treatment is based on the underlying or the presumptive cause:

(i)   drug overdose — lavage, antidote, dialysis (if drug is dialysable),

(ii)   drug withdrawal — re-introduction, alternative drug,

(iii) systemic sepsis — empirical antibiotic based on presumed source of sepsis,

(iv) CNS infection — IV acyclovir for encephalitis and IV antibiotic for meningitis,

(v)   respiratory failure (either hypoxemia or hypercapnia) — oxygen supplementation $\pm$ ventilatory support.

ANAEMIA
KUEH YAN KOON

Definition
Hb < 13.0 g/dL in adult men; Hb < 12.0 g/dL in adult women. Mild anaemia Hb > 10 g/dL; moderate anaemia Hb 7–10 g/dL; severe anaemia Hb < 7 g/dL.

Anaemia is a common problem and apart from overt gastrointestinal bleeding, the cause is often obscure.

Clinical evaluation
Look for clinical clues for the cause of anaemia from history and physical examination.

1. History: recent onset symptoms — likely an acquired disorder; chronic or episodic — likely a congenital disorder; melena, menorrhagia, pica — iron deficiency; episodic jaundice — haemolytic disorder; food fads/vegetarian — isolated or multiple deficiencies; chronic illness — impaired iron re-utilisation; chemical/radiation exposure — bone marrow injury.
2. Physical: jaundice ± splenomegaly — hemolytic disorder; koilonychia, gum hypertrophy — severe iron deficiency; lymphadenopathy/hepatosplenomegaly/cachexia — neoplastic process; smooth red tongue, signs of subacute combined degeneration — vitamin B12 deficiency; edentulous elderly — multiple deficiencies especially folate.

Investigations
1. FBC (include platelet count) and differential count, **peripheral blood film** for morphological classification of RBCs, PT and PTT (exclude bleeding), reticulocyte count (differentiate between a production problem and peripheral cause), electrolytes, urea and creatinine, LFT.
2. CXR if indicated.
3. GI endoscopy if blood loss obvious or suspected.

PBF description	Diagnostic schema for anaemia
Normochromic, normocytic RBCs	– Screen for systemic illness – Exclude combined deficiencies (Fe/folate/B12) – If above excluded and anaemia severe, examine bone marrow
Microcytic RBCs with (a) Hypochromia	– Confirm Fe deficiency (serum ferritin low, serum Fe/TIBC × 100% < 15%) – Thorough search for source of chronic blood loss — gastrointestinal/gynaecological – Where pertinent, exclude chronic intravascular haemolysis due to paroxysmal nocturnal haemoglobinuria (urine haemosiderinuria, Ham's test) or prosthetic heart valve
(b) Target cells ± basophilic stippling	– Screen for α or β thalassemia
Macrocytic RBCs with (a) Polychromiasia ± spherocytes	Confirm presence of haemolysis (increased reticulocytes, unconjugated bilirubin, LDH) then define specific haemolytic process e.g. AIHA, G6PD deficiency, hereditary spherocytosis, etc.
(b) Ovalocytes and hypersegmented neutrophils	Determine Vitamin B12 and folate levels: – low folate, exclude nutritional cause and malabsorption – B12 low, exclude nutritional cause, postgastrectomy deficiency of intrinsic factor – both folate and B12 low, exclude nutritional cause and malabsorption
(c) Varying degrees of poikilocytosis and normal folate and B12 levels	Bone marrow examination with cytogenetics to exclude myelodysplastic syndrome
(d) Target cells	Screen for chronic liver disease

PBF description	Diagnostic schema for anaemia
Dimorphic RBCs (mixed normocytic/ normochromic and microcytic/hypochromic RBCs)	
(a) With poikilocytosis	Exclude sideroblastic anaemia (increased Fe saturation, marrow ringed sideroblasts ± marrow cytogenetic derangements
(b) Without poikilocytosis	History of recent packed cell transfusion, Fe therapy for iron deficiency. If history negative, proceed as for (a) to exclude sideroblastic anaemial

The most common PBF for patients with mild to moderate anaemia is normochromic normocytic RBCs. When anaemia is mild and a chronic illness is evident, there is no need to go beyond establishing normal serum levels of haematinics. However, if anaemia is moderate or severe and serum haematinic levels are normal, a bone marrow examination is mandatory.

HYPOTENSION AND SHOCK
LEE KANG HOE

Introduction
When hypotension occurs, there is a fall in the perfusion pressure of various organs. This will lead to organ dysfunction and eventually failure, if the hypotension is prolonged. This will then ultimately lead to death if not corrected. Our body will attempt to maintain central perfusion pressure by vasoconstricting flow to "non-vital" areas, and thus when systemic hypotension occurs, the patient is in danger. It is thus important to detect the signs for early shock (tachycardia, cool peripheries, oliguria, mental obtundation) before it becomes overt.

Clinical evaluation
1. History and physical looking for features of shock (tachycardia, chest pain, dyspnoea, cool peripheries, oliguria, mental obtundation) and causes. Document vitals. Look for bleeding.
2. Important to establish the cause of hypotension:
   (i) Low cardiac output: inadequate preload (hemorrhage, severe dehydration, pericardial restriction); cardiac failure (infarction/ischemia, hypertensive heart, cardiomyopathy, arrhythmia, valvular heart disease).
   (ii) Low systemic vascular resistance: sepsis, anaphylaxis, liver failure, pancreatitis, spinal shock, thyrotoxicosis.

Investigations
1. FBC, electrolytes, urea and creatinine, liver function test, DIC screen, ABG, CK, CKMB, X-match, lactate, amylase (as indicated).
2. Cultures if sepsis suspected.
3. Imaging: CXR, and depending on symptoms.
4. ECG.

Management

Shock is a medical emergency. Treatment should be rapid and the shock reversed as quickly as possible.

1. Two large IV peripheral lines.
2. Supplemental oxygen (high flow).
3. Catheterise the bladder.
4. Run fluids fast — isotonic crystalloids (normal saline or Ringer's lactate) or colloids (Gelafundin, Haesteril 6% or PPF 4.5%). Give at least 2 litres, unless the patient is overloaded or there is concern of heart failure.
5. Consider central pressure monitoring (CVP or PA catheter) if hypotension still evident.
6. ICU admission may be desirable.
7. Start inotrope (Dopamine — 1 to 20 µg/kg/min or Noradrenaline — 0 to 2 µg/kg/min).
8. Give more fluids if indicated by central monitoring.
9. Consider intubation.
10. Invasive blood pressure monitoring.
11. Give blood if hemoglobin < 10 g/dl. Correct coagulopathy if bleeding.
12. Always treat the underlying cause of hypotension (e.g. antibiotics ± drainage for sepsis)
13. Re-evaluate the progress of treatment (mental status, urine output, ECG, resolution of acidosis)
14. Other inotropes to consider — adrenaline or dobutamine if cardiac output low despite adequate preload (PAWP 15 to 20 mmHg).
15. IABP for acute AMI, or acute MR or VSD from ischemia.
16. Consider thrombolysis or thrombectomy for severe PE.

FEVER AND RASH

CHAN HENG LEONG and WONG SOON TEE

Introduction

Three main groups of causes: infections, drug reactions, or connective tissue disorders.

Clinical evaluation

1. History: recent exposure to others with infectious diseases; sexual exposure; and detailed drug history including information from GP.
2. Accurate morphological diagnosis of the rash critical in **differential diagnosis**.

Erythematous/exanthematous eruption:

   (i) Infections — Viral infections (measles (Koplik's spots), rubella, infectious mononucleosis, dengue, HIV infection (conversion)); Bacterial infections (toxic shock syndrome, secondary syphilis)
   (ii) Non-infectious disorders — exanthematic drug reactions; erythema multiforme; systemic lupus erythematosus

Purpuric eruptions:

   (i) Life-threatening infections (rapid deterioration, often with shock, DIC, gangrene) — meningococcal septicaemia (maculopapular rash may be present before ecchymoses); rickettsial infection; scrub typhus (eschar); listeria; staphyloccocus; streptococcus pneumonia; infective endocarditis; malaria; dengue.
   (ii) Non-infectious disorders — leucocytoclastic vasculitis; Henoch-Schonlein purpura; acute SLE; drug reactions.

Vesiculo-pustular eruptions:

   (i) Infections — Viral infections (varicella, herpes zoster, herpes simplex); Bacterial infections (secondary bacterial infection of vesicles, staphylococcal scalded skin syndrome).

   (ii) Non-infectious disorders — drug reactions (Stevens-Johnson syndrome/Toxic epidermal necrolysis); pustular psoriasis; pemphigus/pemphigoid.

Nodular lesions:
   (i)   Erythematous — erythema nodosum.
   (ii) Non-erythematous — fungal (e.g. candida); mycobacteria (TB or atypical) infection; lymphoma.

Differential diagnoses in specific clinical situations:
   (i)   Pustules associated with arthralgias — gonococcaemia; meningoccocaemia; infective endocarditis; Behcet's syndrome.
   (ii) Meningitis associated with rash: Purpura — meningococcus, echovirus 9, coxsackie, leptospira, Staphylococcus aureus, acute HIV; Herpes progenitalis or labialis — Herpes simplex; Papulonodular — cryptococcus.
   (iii) Encephalitis associated with rash — Herpes zoster/simplex, measles, enterovirus.

CARDIOLOGY

CARDIOPULMONARY RESUSCITATION
NG WAI LIN

In the event of cardiac arrest, the first thing to do is to remain calm and not to panic. However, there must be a sense of urgency, and resuscitation should commence immediately as cerebral damage is likely to occur within minutes. There should be a designated leader who coordinates the resuscitation.

1. The first thing to do is to CONFIRM the diagnosis of cardiac arrest (unconscious, cyanotic, pulseless with no heart sound).
2. Activate code team (if present in hospital).
3. Basic cardiac life support should commence immediately (A(airway), B(breathing) (circulation)).
4. ECG leads should be attached to determine the underlying rhythm: pulseless VT, VFib, PEA (Pulseless electrical activity), asystole, or an agonal. Refer to the algorithms for specific therapies.

    As there are usually several people present in the arrest, different functions are carried out simultaneously rather than in sequence as outlined.
5. Check the airway and respiration. Exclude upper airway obstruction. Remove dentures or food debris. Insert an oropharyngeal airway. Ventilate with bag-valve mask.
6. Obtain multiple peripheral venous access. Sometimes a central venous access is necessary. Drugs can be given through the tracheal tube at double the iv dose if peripheral venous access cannot be obtained.
7. Consider intubation.

Several key points to remember during resuscitation:
1. Do not interrupt basic cardiac life support for more than 10 seconds.
2. Intravenous 1 mg adrenaline should be given every 5 minutes while resuscitation is being carried out.

3. Sodium bicarbonate should not be given routinely except during prolonged resuscitation. Frequency and doses given should be guided by blood pH.
4. Calcium chloride and bicarbonate should not be given the rough the same line.
5. ACLS as outline by the AHA is only a guideline and deviation from this is permissible in individual cases.
6. Apart from BCLS, early defibrillation is the most important manoeuvre and takes precedence over intubation or administration of medication.
7. The other drug worth considering in refractory VT or VF is intravenous amiodarone (300 mg bolus).
8. Consider calcium chloride only if hyperkalaemia, hypocalcaemia or calcium-channel blocker overdose is suspected.
9. Successful resuscitation from cardiac arrest in unwitnessed, prolonged arrest, asystole or electromechanical resuscitation is uncommon.
10. Consider termination of CPR after 15 minutes if there are no further reversible factors to correct, and there is still no return of spontaneous circulation (ROSC).
11. Once ROSC is maintained, consider the requirements for dopamine infusion or lignocaine infusion as indicated.
12. Transfer to ICU/CCU when BP and rhythm is stable for at least 10 minutes.
13. Accompany patient during transport with ECG monitoring, defibrillator, intubation equipment, and drugs.

Algorithms:

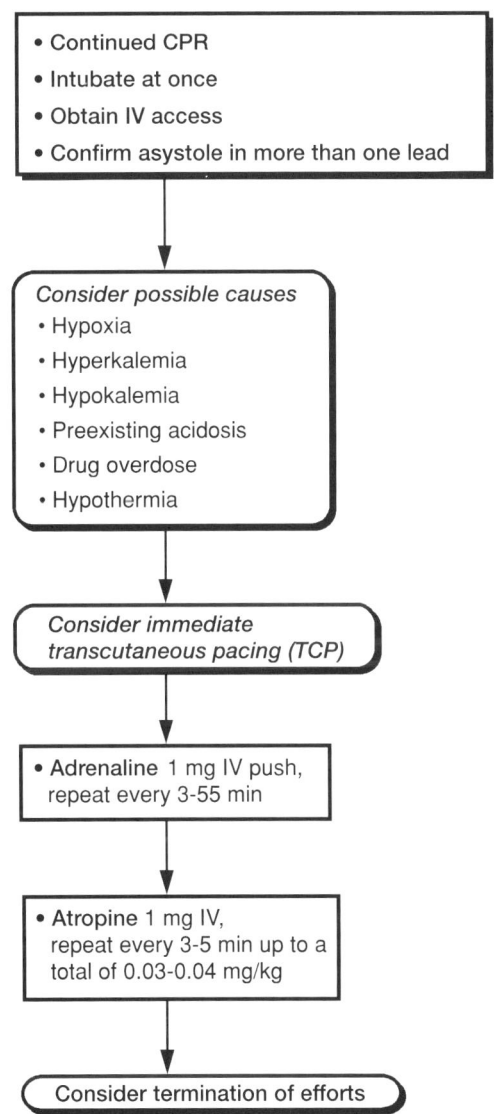

- Continued CPR
- Intubate at once
- Obtain IV access
- Confirm asystole in more than one lead

Consider possible causes
- Hypoxia
- Hyperkalemia
- Hypokalemia
- Preexisting acidosis
- Drug overdose
- Hypothermia

Consider immediate transcutaneous pacing (TCP)

- Adrenaline 1 mg IV push, repeat every 3-55 min

- Atropine 1 mg IV, repeat every 3-5 min up to a total of 0.03-0.04 mg/kg

Consider termination of efforts

Figure 1. Asystole Treatment Algorithm.

23

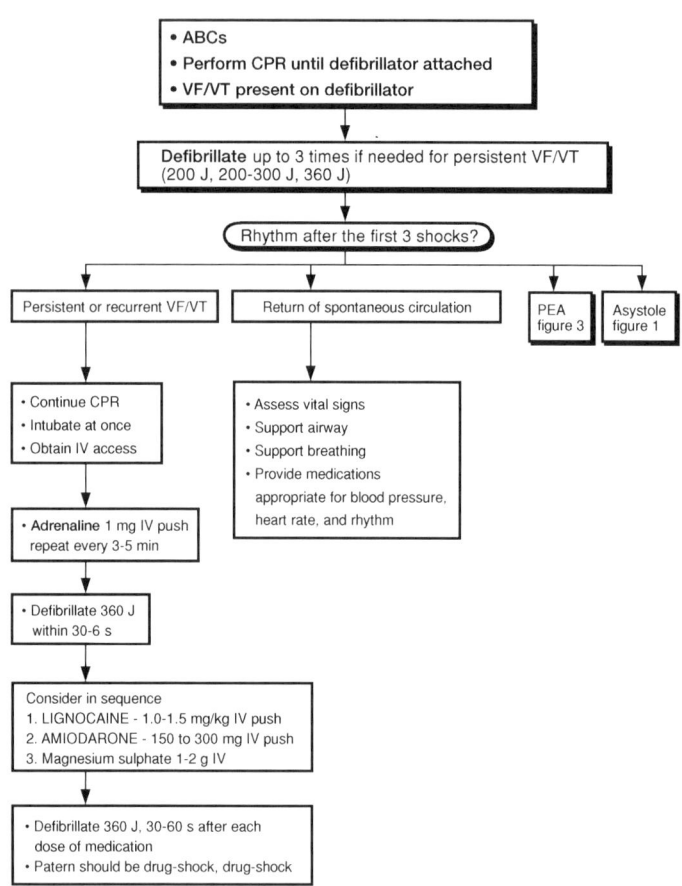

Figure 2. Ventricular Fibrillation/Pulseless Ventricular Tachycardia (VG/VT) Algorithm.

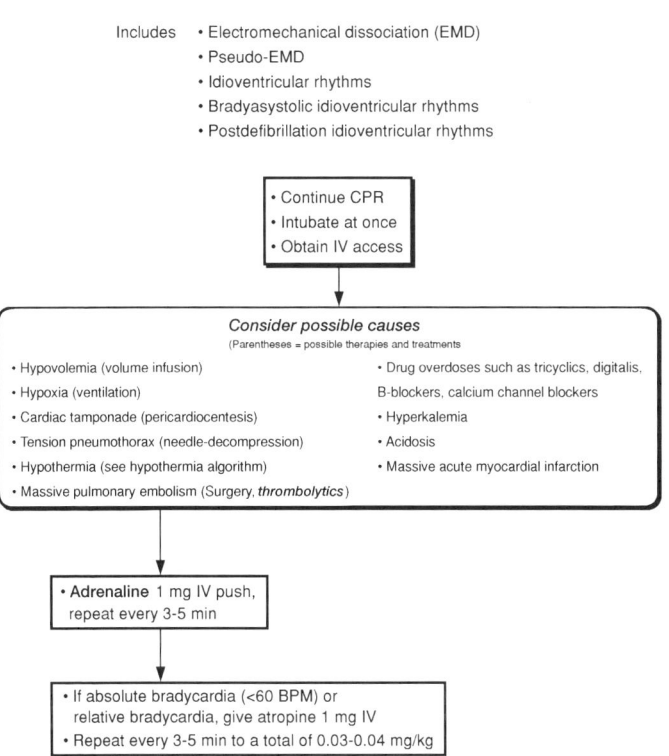

Includes
- Electromechanical dissociation (EMD)
- Pseudo-EMD
- Idioventricular rhythms
- Bradyasystolic idioventricular rhythms
- Postdefibrillation idioventricular rhythms

- Continue CPR
- Intubate at once
- Obtain IV access

Consider possible causes
(Parentheses = possible therapies and treatments)

- Hypovolemia (volume infusion)
- Hypoxia (ventilation)
- Cardiac tamponade (pericardiocentesis)
- Tension pneumothorax (needle-decompression)
- Hypothermia (see hypothermia algorithm)
- Massive pulmonary embolism (Surgery, *thrombolytics*)

- Drug overdoses such as tricyclics, digitalis, B-blockers, calcium channel blockers
- Hyperkalemia
- Acidosis
- Massive acute myocardial infarction

- **Adrenaline** 1 mg IV push, repeat every 3-5 min

- If absolute bradycardia (<60 BPM) or relative bradycardia, give atropine 1 mg IV
- Repeat every 3-5 min to a total of 0.03-0.04 mg/kg

Figure 3. Pulseless Electrical Activity (PEA) Algorithm (Electromechanical Dissociation (EMD)).

ACUTE MYOCARDIAL INFARCTION (AMI)
LING LIENG HSI

Definition
Requires 2 of 3 criteria: 1. History of ischemic chest discomfort, 2. Serial ECGs changes, 3. Rise and fall in serum cardiac markers.

Clinical evaluation
1. Diagnostic considerations:
   (i)   ST-segment elevation and/or Q waves on ECG are highly indicative of AMI, but absent in about 50% of pts. Thus, for the majority of pts, serial cardiac enzyme changes are essential in establishing the diagnosis.
   (ii) Current laboratory tests do not detect AMI within the first 4 hrs with sufficient sensitivity to impact on emergency treatment. Acute management of AMI is thus based principally on history and ECG.
   (iii) Not every ST-elevation AMI evolves into a Q wave AMI. Therefore, the clinical distinction between unstable angina, Q and non-Q AMI can only be made retrospectively after serial ECGs and serum cardiac markers have been obtained.
   (iv) Certain subgps may present with atypical symptoms. In the elderly, shortness of breath more frequent than ischemic chest pain.

2. Differential diagnoses:
   (i)   Clinical: aortic dissection — inferior AMI is a classic association, acute pericarditis, acute myocarditis, spontaneous pneumothorax, pulmonary embolism.
   (ii) ECG: normal variant, acute pericarditis.

   If AMI suspected, but ECG changes non-diagnostic or inapparent:

(i) Examine serial tracings for development of ST elevation.

(ii) Request 2-D echo for regional wall motion abnormalities. Echo is also of particular value for excluding aortic dissection.

Investigations

1. FBC, elcetrolytes, urea and creatinine, CK and CKMB (8 hourly × 3), PT, PTT, Group and save.
2. ECG — do right-sided leads as well if inferior AMI looking for RV infarct (ST elevation in V4R), 8 hourly × 3.
3. CXR.
4. 2D-echo as indicated.

Management

1. High risk indicators: previous AMI, persistent ischemic chest pain, CHF, hypotension, heart block, hemodynamically compromising ventricular arrhythmias. Low risk pts can be transferred out of CCU within 24–36 hours.

2. General measures: Establish IV access; ECG monitoring; supplemental oxygen (pulse oximetry monitoring is useful) — may require ventilation; analgesia — control pain with reperfusion therapy, oxygen, nitrates and beta-blockers, give morphine as well (IV 2–4 mg every 5 minutes till pain relieved); bed rest — short-term; anxiolytics only if required (lorazepam 0.5–1 mg nocte); stool softener — senna 2 tabs nocte.

3. Aspirin — administer to all pts: 300 mg chewed on admission (for rapid absorption), then 100 mg (enteric coated) daily. Use ticlopidine 250 mg daily if aspirin contraindicated.

4. Thrombolytic agent — Pts treated within 12 hours who are eligible for thrombolytics should receive expeditiously either accelerated (frontloaded) tPA or SK (or be considered for primary PTCA).

Indications:

(i) ECG: ST elevation (> 0.1 mV in ≥ 2 contiguous leads), or new BBB,

(ii) Time to therapy < 6 hrs. Small benefit after 12–24 hrs, but consider thrombolysis if ongoing ischemic pain and extensive ST elevation.

(iii) Age < 75 yrs – age > 75 not a contraindication but a higher risk of ICH expected.

(iv) Consider thrombolysis when above criteria absent but there is: giant, hyperacute T waves without ST-segment elevation (early phase AMI), or acute posterior infarction with ST depression in V1-V4 (circumflex artery occlusion).

5. Administration:

(i) Accelerated tPA — IV 15 mg bolus, then 50 mg over 30 min and 35 mg over 60 min. Dose of tPA should be adjusted downward for pts < 67 kg.

(ii) SK — IV 1.5 MU over 60 min.

6. Choice of thrombolytics: Accelerated tPA with IV heparin is the most effective therapy for achieving early coronary reperfusion but substantially more expensive and carries greater risk of ICH. Reasonable to use tPA for pts at moderate to high risk and SK for pts at low to moderate risk. Contraindications for SK use — usage in last 1 year, and proven allergy.

7. If persistent pain following thrombolysis, consider:

(i) Recurrent myocardial ischemia — Use IV beta-blocker and IV GTN. May consider readministration of tPA if recurrent ST elevation, or emergent coronary angiography KIV revascularisation

(ii) Acute pericarditis — probably not responsible for chest discomfort in first 24 hrs. Use aspirin (up to 600 mg 4–6 hrly).

(iii) Impending myocardial rupture — request 2-D echo.

8. Beta-blockers for:

(i) All pts without specific contraindications,

(ii) Continuing or recurrent ischemic pain,

(iii) Tachyarrhythmias e.g. AF with rapid ventricular response.

Use short acting drugs if concern about hemodynamic stability or tolerance, e.g. metoprolol.

If IV use considered, give metoprolol IV 15 mg (2.5–5 mg every 2–5 min) followed by oral 50 mg BID for 1 day and then 100 mg BID or atenolol IV 2.5–5.0 mg over 2 min to total of 10 mg in 10–15 min followed by oral 100 mg daily. Aim for SBP < 100 mm Hg and HR < 50 bpm. Usual contraindications.

9. Nitrates may be used for 24–48 hrs in pts with CHF, persistent or recurrent ischemia, or hypertension. Use IV GTN which allows precise control and rapid termination of effect in the event of adverse effects. Pump-controlled infusion of 5 µg/min, increase by 5 µg/min q 10 min while carefully monitoring BP, HR and clinical response. Do not exceed >200 µg/min. When using IV GTN for 24–48 hours continuously, drug tolerance may occur. Titrate to abolish symptoms, decrease in MAP by 10% in normotensive pts or 30% in hypertensive pts, without allowing SBP to fall below 90 mmHg (or MAP < 80 mmHg).

10. IV Heparin with tPA. Administer 70 IU/kg bolus after the end of tPA followed by 15 IU/kg/hr. Check aPTT 4–6 hours after initiating therapy or changing dose. Keep aPTT between 50 to 75 seconds (or 1.5–2.0 × control).

Maintain IV heparin for > 48 hours only if high-risk pts or for prophylaxis of systemic or venous thromboembolism (see following).

11. IV Heparin for prevention of systemic embolism (regardless of thrombolytic agent used) in pts with large, anterior AMI, LV thrombus by echocardiography, previous embolic event, or AF.

12. Prevention of DVT in pts at high risk. Give s/c heparin 5000–7500 units BID.

13. ACE inhibitors for anterior AMI, previous AMI, CHF, tachycardia, and LV ejection fraction <40%. Usual

contraindications. Administer within first 24 hours, after completion of thrombolytic therapy and stabilization of BP. Begin with low dose (e.g. captopril 6.25 mg) and increase steadily to achieve full dose within 24–48 hrs.

14. Calcium channel blockers — Verapamil and diltiazem may reduce incidence of reinfarction in pts with first non-Q wave AMI or first inferior AMI without LV dysfunction or pulmonary congestion, but their benefit beyond that of beta-blockers and aspirin is unclear.

15. Arrhythmias (see relevant chapters). Ventricular arrhythmias not requiring treatment: isolated PVCs or couplets, idioventricular rhythm, non-sustained VT (< 5 beats).

16. Indications for temporary cardiac pacing: asystole, 3rd-degree AV block (anterior AMI, wide escape QRS complex, or inferior AMI with no response to atropine), bilateral BBB (alternating BBB, RBBB with alternating LAFB/LPFB), bifascicular block (RBBB + LAFB/LPFB or LBBB) with first-degree AV block, type II AV block, regardless of AMI location, and all other symptomatic bradycardias not responding promptly to atropine.

17. Consider pacing if: RBBB and LAFB or LPFB (new or indeterminate), RBBB with first-degree AV block, LBBB — new or indeterminate, incessant VT (overdrive pacing), or recurrent sinus pauses (> 3 seconds) not responsive to atropine.

18. A transvenous pacing electrode should be placed in pts who require ongoing pacing and in those

19. Beware of MR from papillary muscle rupture, VSD, LV free wall rupture for sudden deteriorations and heart failure.

20. In RV AMI the treatment for hypotension is to volume load. Consider PA catheter to guide volume resuscitation.

21. IABP may help in severe heart failure as a bridge to revascularisation.

22. Primary PTCA — when thrombolytic therapy is absolutely contraindicated.

23. Indications for early coronary angiography following AMI:
    (i)   Stuttering episodes of spontaneous or induced ischemia,
    (ii) Postinfarction angina,
    (iii) Cardiogenic shock,
    (iv) CHF or noninvasive evidence of LV systolic dysfunction.

DIAGNOSIS AND MANAGEMENT OF COMMON ARRHYTHMIAS
NG KHENG SIANG

Tachyarrhythmias may be:
(i) supraventricular, arising from the atria or around the A-V node, or
(ii) ventricular, arising from below the A-V node.
They may adversely affect the haemodynamic perform-ance of the heart (loss of atrial transport, increase in myocardial oxygen requirement or loss of organised ventricular contraction). Some are benign and do not warrant treatment, e.g. atrial or ventricular extrasystole. Others can be life-threatening and thereby mandate quick action (e.g. ventricular fibrillation).
   Bradyarrythmias may allow escape tachyarrhythmias or lead to hypotension and asystole.

Clinical evaluation
1. Establish heart rate (regularity), BP, mental status, pres-ence of chest pain.
2. Review medications (pro-arrhythmic agents)

Investigation
1. Perform ECG (determine QRS length: < 0.12 secs con-sidered narrow complex).
2. Check electrolytes (include magnesium, and calcium)

Management
A. Narrow complex tachycardia — HR > 150 bpm. Some patients may be asymptomatic and appear comfortable, while others may appear hypotensive and highly distressed.

1. Supraventricular tachycardia — atrioventricular nodal reentrant or atrioventricular reciprocating
2. Atrial tachycardia;

3. Atrial flutter;
4. Atrial fibrillation.

Treatment aimed at restoring sinus rhythm.
1. Carotid sinus massage. Rub the right carotid artery (sinus) for 5–6 seconds at a time. Switch to the left carotid sinus if the right fails. Listen first for a carotid bruit (especially elderly), to avoid precipitating a stroke.
2. iv adenosine triphosphate (ATP). Quick bolus. Start with 6 mg. Increase by 3 mg until 24 mg. Short half-life of 2–3 seconds. Transient A-V block. Patients often complain of an unpleasant but fleeting sensation within the head or chest. Effective for supraventricular tachycardia, sinus node reentrant tachycardia and certain forms of atrial tachycardia, but does not work for atrial flutter or fibrillation. Diagnostic tool for narrow complex tachycardia, by unmasking the P waves.
3. Intravenous verapamil. Start with a slow bolus dose of 5 mg, to be repeated at 5 minute intervals till a maximum cumulative dose of 20 mg. Contraindicated if the patient is hypotensive (can consider giving iv calcium first) or in heart failure. It will not terminate atrial flutter or tachycardia but will slow the ventricular response.
4. Other drugs that may be considered include: iv digoxin 0.25 mg to 1 mg (if not given previously); iv propranolol 1 mg to 10 mg; iv flecainide 50 mg to 100 mg; iv disopyramide 50 mg to 150 mg; iv amiodarone 150 mg.
5. DC cardioversion for those resistant to drug therapy, or those with haemodynamic. Atrial flutter may be successfully cardioverted using as little as 25 J while atrial fibrillation or tachycardia will generally require at least 100 J. Set to synchronised mode to reduce the risk of inducing VF.
6. Alternatively, the patient may be transferred to the CCU for an attempt at overdrive pacing.

B. Wide complex tachycardia — Important to identify ventricular tachycardia; potentially fatal arrhythmia. ECG criteria in favour of diagnosis: AV dissociation; presence of captured or fusion beats; superior axis, especially if the axis is normal during sinus rhythm; if RBBB pattern — monophasic R wave in V1, triphasic R wave with R > R', ie. taller left rabbit ear, rS or QS pattern in V5, V6; if LBBB pattern — small but fat r wave in V1, rS > 110 ms duration. If in doubt, treat the arrhythmia as a VT until proven otherwise.

1. Ventricular tachycardia;
2. Supraventricular tachycardia with aberrancy;
3. Sinus tachycardia with preexisting bundle branch block;
4. Preexcited tachycardia (utilises an accessory pathway for antegrade conduction)

Management depends on clinical and haemodynamic status of the patient:
1. In the event of haemodynamic collapse, when the patient is already unconscious, cardiovert with 200 J. If not successful, repeat with 200 J and then increase to 300 J. If still unsuccessful, intubate and proceed as in ACLS protocol.
2. Hypotensive but conscious patient: ensure adequate sedation of the patient with iv midazolam or propofol prior to cardioversion. Synchronize cardioversion (200 J).
3. Conscious patient who is haemodynamically stable: chemical cardioversion may be attempted. See algorithm in CPR chapter. If drug therapy fails, the patient can be transferred to the CCU for semi-emergency cardioversion or overdrive pacing.

C. Atrial fibrillation in WPW — irregularly irregular wide complex tachyarrhythmia.

Manage as for VT. Use iv procainamide, disopyramide or flecainide. They act by interrupting conduction down the accessory pathway.

D. Bradyarrhythmias — Dysfunction of the sino-atrial node, atrioventricular node or the His-Purkinje system. Generally not necessary to treat unless there is giddiness, near syncope, syncope, hypotension, or congestive heart failure. Long term management requires a permanent pacemaker. Until this can be done, drugs or temporary cardiac pacing may be required as an interim emergency measure.

1. Sick sinus syndrome: inappropriate sinus bradycardia; sino-atrial nodal exit block or pause; bradytachy syndrome.
2. AV block: AV nodal Wenckebach; Mobitz type II AV block; complete heart block; junctional bradycardia.

Management

(i)   IV atropine. Start with IV 0.3 mg and repeat until a desirable heart rate is achieved. Do not exceed 2.1 mg. Will not work for infra-Hisian blocks or denervated hearts (heart transplant).

(ii) Isoprenaline. Dilute 0.2 mg in 20 ml normal saline and infuse at 1–3 (g/min according to the heart rate response. BP may fall from peripheral vasodilation and venous pooling.

(iii) Cardiac pacing. Absolute indications: complete heart block with hypotension, cardiac failure and mental obtundation; alternating right and left bundle branch blocks; asystolic pause of at least 3 secs with giddiness or syncope; QT prolongation with torsades de pointes. Relative indications: complete heart block without hypotension, cardiac failure or mental obtundation; bifascicular or trifascicular block; overdrive pacing of refractory tachycardias. Emergency pacing can be effected transcutaneously or transvenously.

CONGESTIVE HEART FAILURE
LIM YEAN TENG

Pathophysiology

Congestive Heart Failure: when cardiac output is inadequate to maintain forward flow at a rate commensurate with requirements of the body, or is only able to do so at an elevated filling pressure.

(Alternative definition — a complex clinical syndrome characterised by abnormalities of left ventricular function and neuro-hormonal regulation, which are accompanied by reduced effort tolerance, fluid retention, and reduced longevity.)

Clinical evaluation

1. Assessment: hemodynamic, respiratory, mental status (check vital signs).
2. Look for causes: ischaemia/infarction, arrhythmia, murmurs, thyrotoxicosis, bacterial endocarditis, drugs (β-blocker).
3. Differential diagnoses: pericardial disease, cor pulmonale, fluid-overload states (renal failure, liver cirrhosis, protein-losing enteropathy).

Investigations

1. ECG — 'q' waves, LVH, "Goldberger's" triad (Cardiomyopathy — small limb leads but tall chest leads voltages, with poor R wave progression in anterior chest leads), cardiac arrhythmias (e.g. atrial fibrillation).
2. CXR — cardiomegaly, and pulmonary congestion pleural effusion.
3. Blood investigations: ABG, FBC, electrolytes, urea and creatinine, cardiac enzymes, liver enzymes.
4. 2D-Echo — assess LV function, and causes of heart failure.

Management

1. Rest the patient in bed. Restrict fluid and salt intake.
2. Administer oxygen by nasal prong (e.g. 4L/min) or face-mask (e.g. 40%).
3. Diuretics (alleviate symptoms). For rapid effect, IV frusemide 40 to 80 mg bolus, or bumetanide 1mg bolus. Subsequent dose may be oral or parenteral.
4. ACE-inhibitors if there is left ventricular systolic dysfunction and absence of contraindications. Reduces morbidity and mortality. Captopril 6.25 mg to 12.5 mg bid or tid and increase as tolerated. Other ACE-inhibitors can be employed.
5. Digoxin will improve symptoms even in those with sinus rhythm.
6. Investigate precipitating factors (e.g. non-compliance with medicine/fluid or salt restriction/anaemia, etc.), and correct them.
7. Patients with low BP/cardiogenic shock should be managed in ICU for inotropic support, invasive monitoring, and mechanical ventilation. IABP or other ventricular assist devices may be an important bridge for those suitable for cardiac transplantation.
8. Look for reversible ischaemia (hibernating myocardium). Consider early revascularisation.

PULMONARY EMBOLISM
LIM TAI TIAN and LEE KANG HOE

Pathophysiology

Embolus leads to hypoxemia and hemodynamic compromise. Shunt develops from collapsed alveolus in ischemic areas, and potentially through intra-cardiac shunting through patent foramen ovales from pulmonary hypertension. Cardiac output is compromised and mixed venous saturation falls as another mechanism of arterial oxygen desaturation. A big saddle embolus will cause acute right-sided ventricular failure with consequent decrease in cardiac output and hence, hemodynamic collapse. Occasionally, pulmonary infarction occurs if the bronchial circulation is also compromised — this will lead to hemoptysis and pleurisy.

Clinical evaluation

1. Look for chest pain (pleuritic nature), cough (with hemoptysis), sudden dyspnoea (cyanosis, tachypnoea), associated DVT.
2. Assess hemodynamic status (HR, BP, perfusion state) and respiratory status (signs of fatigue, oxygenation).
3. Document presence of risk factors: bed-bound patient, especially 1 week after surgery (high-risk — orthopaedic cases); previous thromboembolic disease; malignancy; obesity; heart failure.

Investigations

1. Blood investigations: ABG (hypoxemia with respiratory alkalosis — may be normal), FBC, DIVC screen (look for raised D-dimers — high sensitivity but low specificity), Protein C and S, anti-thrombin III levels.
2. ECG (changes only in massive embolisation: lead I: prominent S wave; lead III: large Q wave; inverted T wave; V1-V4: T wave inversion). Classical S1Q3T3 pattern seen in 12%.

3. Imaging: CXR (peripheral wedge-shaped opacity if pulmonary infarction), V/Q scan (high probability — accuracy of 96%), CT thorax (spiral — peripheral emboli may be missed), Duplex scan of lower limbs, Pulmonary angiogram.

(Gold standard pulmonary angiogram. CT thorax useful for proximal lesions. V/Q scan difficult to interpret in presence of abnormal chest radiograph.)

Diagnosis

Clinical and imaging. May require treatment if clinical suspicion is high before imaging if delayed.

Management

1. Prevention — mobilise as soon as possible. Subcutaneous heparin (Heparin 5000 units bid sc or Fraxiparine 0.3 ml om sc) or even low dose warfarin in high-risk patients. Prevent dehydration.
2. If severely ill — consider embolectomy (if thrombolysis contraindicated, but mortality high), or even thrombolysis (SK 250,000 IU over 30 minutes then 100,000 units/hr over 24 hours; rt-PA 10 mg bolus, followed by 90 mg over 2 hours).
3. Anticoagulation — heparin followed by warfarin. IV heparin 5000 units bolus, followed by 1500 units/hr (reduce or increase according to body weight). Check PTT in 4 to 6 hours, Adjust to achieve PTT 2.5 times normal. Contraindicated if bleeding risk high or active bleeding present — may then consider vena caval filter. Other option: low molecular weight heparin (fraxiparine 0.4 ml bd sc for weight <50 kg, 0.5 ml bd sc for 50 to 65 kg, and 0.6 ml for >65 kg). Warfarin required for 6 months — start oral warfarin when patient stable and there is little risk for surgical intervention.
4. Supportive measures: supplemental oxygen, pain-relief, fluid resuscitation and inotropes.

HYPERTENSIVE EMERGENCIES AND URGENCIES
CHIA BOON LOCK

Definition
Hypertensive emergency: LIFE-THREATENING, severe hypertension (diastolic BP usually ≥ 120 to 130 mmHg) associated with acute, progressing target organ disease and requiring prompt BP reduction. Treatment usually in an ICU setting.

Hypertensive urgency: severe hypertension ($\geq 230/130$ mmHg), but without acute target organ damage. If fundal exudates/haemorrhages or papilloedema are also present, diagnose accelerated or malignant hypertension respectively. In hypertensive urgency, BP should be reduced within 24 hours. This is usually carried out on an outpatient basis.

Clinical evaluation
1. Careful history.
2. Examine for target organ damage in the optic fundi, central nervous system, and cardiovascular system. E.g. focal neurologic signs, confusion, coma, heart failure.

Investigations
1. ECG, FBC, electrolytes, urea and creatinine, urine analysis, CXR.
2. CT head or echocardiography may be required if hypertensive neurologic emergencies or aortic dissection are diagnosed respectively.

Management
Table 1 is a list of the drugs that are commonly used. The two most urgent indications for an immediate reduction in BP are hypertensive encephalopathy and aortic dissection. The recommended time taken for the target BP to be achieved

varies widely from several minutes to several hours, depending on the clinical diagnosis.

1. Hypertensive emergencies (Mainly managed in ICU/CCU)

A. Neurological — In neurological hypertensive emergencies, the target BP is approximately 160–180/100–110 mmHg with no greater than a 25% reduction of the mean arterial pressure (MAP). This should be achieved gradually over several hours.

Hypertensive Encephalopathy.
(i)   Admit to ICU.
(ii) IV nitroprusside infusion is the drug of choice, (alternative IV diaxozide).
(iii) Lower BP to the target level within 1–3 hours.
(iv) Start oral hypotensives as well to overlap with nitroprusside.

Subarachnoid Haemorrhage.
(i)   Admit to ICU.
(ii) IV (or oral) nimodipine infusion is drug of choice.
(iii) Lower to target BP within 6 to 12 hours.

Hypertensive intracerebral Haemorrhage.
(i)   Treatment of BP controversial (prognosis poor).
(ii) Oral or sublingual nifedipine (10 mg) may be used.

B. Cardiovascular

Hypertensive Heart Failure (Pulmonary Oedema).
(i)   Admit to CCU if the BP is $\geq$ 230/120–130 mmHg.
(ii) Lower BP quickly to near normal levels with IV nitroprusside infusion.
(iii) Give IV frusemide and other routine measures for acute pulmonary oedema (refer *).

Aortic Dissection.

(i) Admit to CCU.

(ii) Confirm diagnosis (usually by transesophageal echo-cardiography).

(iii) Lower BP within 15 to 30 minutes to systolic 100–120 mmHg and a MAP ≤ 80 mmHg with IV nitroprusside infusion.

(iv) IV propranolol (1–10 mg slowly till heart rate around 60/min) — beneficial negative inotropic effect and reduces shearing force of systolic contraction.

(v) Once the BP is controlled, surgery must be considered in types I and II whilst medical therapy is recommended in type III aortic dissection.

Unstable Angina and Acute Myocardial Infarction.

(i) Admit to CCU.

(ii) Give IV GTN infusion (5-100 µg/min)to lower BP gradually until symptomatic improvement or diastolic BP is around 100 mmHg.

(iii) IV nitroprusside infusion for refractory cases.

C. Others

Eclampsia.

Treated by obstetrician. IV hydralazine (0.1–0.5 mg/min) infusion is the drug of choice.

Phaechromocytoma.

(i) Either miniboluses of phentolamine mesylate (2–5 mg every 5 minutes) or a continuous IV infusion.

(ii) IV labetalol can also be used.

Acute Renal Insufficiency.

IV hydralazine or labetalol infusion is recommended.

2. Hypertensive urgencies

(i) Begin treatment in the emergency department (nifedipine (10 mg sublingually or orally) — some controversy, alternative is felodipine (5–10 mg) or captopril (25 mg))

(ii) Reduce BP to 150–170/100–110 mmHg in a few hours, observe in A & E.

(iii) If response unsatisfactory, admit for further treatment. Otherwise, continue medication as outpatient with early review.

(iv) Admit accelerated/malignant hypertension.

(v) Evaluate renal function and underlying causes.

Table 1

Name	Dose
Sodium Nitroprusside	0.3–10 µg/kg/min. (IV infusion). Usual dose needed 3 µg/kg/min
Nitroglycerine	5–100 µg/min (IV infusion)
Diaxozide	IV boluses of 50 to 100 mg
Hydralazine	IV 0.1–0.5 mg/min (IV infusion)
Labetalol	IV boluses of 20–80 mg (every 10 minutes)
Phentolamine	IV boluses of 2–5 mg

PULMONARY

ACUTE ASTHMA
TAN WAN CHENG

Definition
Exacerbations of asthma (asthma attacks/acute asthma) are episodes of progressively worsening shortness of breath, cough, wheezing, or chest tightness, or some combination of these symptoms.

Clinical evaluation
1. Assess severity (Chart 1). Attack is graded severe if the patient has a lack of response to initial treatment; if the condition deteriorates or if the patient is a high-risk for near-death.
2. Look for high-risk factors: receiving current/recent systemic corticosteroids, recurrent hospitalisation/ER visits, psychiatric disease, previous near-death asthma attacks, non-compliance with asthma medication.
3. Causes for exacerbations: exposure to allergen, infections (URTI), withdrawal of medication.

Management
1. Relieve airflow obstruction quickly. Nebulised bronchodilators — every 20 minutes for 1 hour.
2. Relieve hypoxaemia — supplemental oxygen (high-flow).
3. Restore lung function — systemic steroids (IV hydrocortisone 100 to 200 mg).
4. If severe and poor response within 1 hour, consider iv aminophylline, and subcutaneous or intramuscular beta$_2$-agonist or adrenaline.
5. Patients requiring vigilant attention: inadequate improvement within 1–2 hours of bronchodilator treatment; no improvement after 2–6 hours of systemic steroids; persistent severe airflow limitation (PEFR <40% predicted); further clinical deterioration in speech, respiratory rate, mental state; Past history of "near-death" (previous ICU admission).

6. If patient continues to deteriorate with $PaCO_2$ > 50 mmHg and pH < 7.3, along with worsening mentation, consider ICU admission and mechanical ventilation (continue nebulisation).
7. Ventilated patients should be sedated (midazolam or propofol) and paralysed (vecuronium or atracurium — beware of histamine release if given too quickly) — be alert for barotrauma.
8. Discharge criteria: patient is ambulant comfortably; no nocturnal or early morning awakening needing a bronchodilator; clinical examination is normal or near normal; PEFR or FEV1 >70% predicted after inhaled beta agonist; short-acting inhaled $beta_2$ agonist is needed no more frequently than 4 hourly; ability to use inhaler devices tested to doctor's satisfaction; been on discharge medications for 24 hours.
9. Make plans (medicine and general) for continued care and for prevention of future relapses before discharge.

Dosages and explanations of treatments
1. $Beta_2$ agonists: Combine nebulisation of a short-acting $beta_2$-agonist with an anticholinergic (ipratropium bromide). Dose: 5 mg (1 ml of 0.5% salbutamol respirator solution) with 2 ml of N saline $\pm$ 1 ml (20 drops of 0.025% solution; 0.25 mg) of ipratropium bromide, repeatedly 4–6 hourly. Parenteral $beta_2$-agonist if there is no response to nebulisation treatment. Intramuscular or subcutaneous $beta_2$-agonist may be used. Dose: 0.5 mg salbutamol in 1 ml injected im/sc 4 hourly, or 0.5–1 mg adrenaline (0.5–1 ml of 1:1000 adrenaline) sc/im.
2. Aminophylline: Potential for improvement of respiratory drive, respiratory muscle function, and prolongation of $beta_2$ agonist effect between doses. Do not load when there is a history of prior theophylline ingestion or unsure. Dose: 250 mg–500 mg (0.5 mg/kg/hr) by infusion every 8 hourly.
3. Systemic corticosteroids for moderate or severe exacerbations. Dose: Hydrocortisone 100–200 mg IV 6 hourly or prednisolone 10–60 mg (0.5 mg/kg) daily.

Severity of Asthma Attacks (Chart 1)

Severity	Mild	Moderate	Severe
Breathless	Walking	Talking	At rest
Position	Can lie down	Prefers sitting	Hunched forward
Talks in	Sentences	Phrases	Words
Mental status	May be agitated	Usually agitated	Drowsy
Respiratory rate	Normal	Increased	Increased
Accessory muscles and abdominal-thoraco paradox	No	Yes	Yes
Wheeze	Mild to Moderate	Loud	Decreased
Pulsus paradoxus	Absent (< 10 mmHg)	10–25 mmHg	> 25 mmHg
PEFR	> 80% predicted	60–80%	< 60% (< 100 L/min)
PaO_2 (room air)	Normal	> 60 mmHg	< 60 mmHg
$PaCO_2$	Normal	< 45 mmHg	> 45 mmHg

The presence of several parameters, but not necessarily all, indicate the general classification of the attack.

ACUTE EXACERBATION OF COPD
LIM TOW KEANG

Clinical evaluation
1. Assess vitals — in particular respiratory rate (use of accessory muscles of breathing), presence of cyanosis, mental status.
2. Current complaints: dyspnoea, cough, sputum production, any fever, chest pain.
3. Ask about exercise tolerance and if any home oxygen therapy.
4. Previous history of smoking, old PTB, lung surgery.
5. Look for signs of pneumonia, cervical lymph nodes, pneumothorax, cor pulmonale, clubbing.
6. Check inhaler technique during hospital admission.

Investigations:
1. Blood investigations: ABG, FBC, RP#1, theophylline levels (if previously on).
2. Radiology: CXR.
3. ECG.
4. Sputum cultures.
5. Do not measure peak flows.

Treatment:
1) Oxygen therapy — low levels to correct hypoxemia (mainly V/Q abnormality). Nasal prongs (1 to 2 L/min) or Venturi masks (28 to 30%). Monitor ABGs for hypercapnia and adequate oxygenation ($PaO_2 > 60$ mmHg). Pulse oximetry monitoring is helpful (Keep $SpO_2 > 90\%$).
2) Nebulized $_2$-agonist (salbutamol — 1 ml of 0.5% is 5 mg) with an anti-cholinergic agent (ipratropium bromide — 2 ml of 0.025% is 0.5 mg (40 drops)) may be repeated 2 to 4 hourly according to response. The high flow rates required for nebulisation may be derived from an electrically driven air-compressor. Be careful of using high flow oxygen for nebulisation in hypercapnic patients. In

hypoxemic patients, provide low-flow oxygen via nasal prongs while nebulising with compressed air.

3) Theophyllines — modest clinical efficacy. Do not give an intravenous "push" unless levels are known, especially if there is a history of regular ingestion. Oral theophyllines can be used as a slow-release preparation (TheoDur 200 to 300 mg bid). IV dosing is 0.5 mg/kg/hr. Lower doses should be used in the presence of cor pulmonale, liver failure, and the use of certain drugs (quinolone, erythromycin, verapamil).

4) Corticosteroids — Tailing dose of oral prednisolone starting at 30 to 40 mg per day over 7 to 10 days. Every attempt should be made to stop corticosteroids by 2 weeks. Inhaled steroids are not indicated for acute exacerbations.

5) Antibiotics — not all exacerbations are provoked by intercurrent bacterial infections. If there is increased sputum purulence, the practice is to treat with a course of antibiotics. The main pathogens isolated are Strep pneumonia, Haem influenzae, and Moraxella catarrhalis. As such, the choice of antibiotics can include a second generation cephalosporin (cefuroxime 500 mg bid po), a beta-lactam/beta-lactamase inhibitor (Unasyn ii bid po, Augmentin 375 mg tid), a quinolone (ciprofloxacin 250 mg bid po) or an extended macrolide (Azithromycin, clarithromycin).

6) Cough mixtures — those containing codeine or an opiate may be helpful.

7) Mucolytic agents — flumucil (600 mg om po), bisolvan, nucosolvan — no proven benefit.

8) Respiratory stimulants — doxapram. No influence on outcome and should not be used routinely.

9) Ventilatory support — noninvasive or intubation. A worsening sensorium, increasing $PaCO_2$ and a falling arterial pH (< 7.25) are indicators of treatment failure and the need for ventilatory support. The appropriateness of such support has to be considered carefully. The concern is the inability to wean the patient off mechanical support and the specter of home ventilation.

HEMOPTYSIS
LIM TOW KEANG

Clinical evaluation
1. Assess hemodynamic stability and respiratory status.
2. Distinguish bleeding from nose, mouth or stomach.
3. Attempt to quantify the amount and frequency of hemoptysis. Massive hemoptysis is defined as 200 to 400 mL/day. Even a small amount may be life-threatening, especially in those with heart-lung disease. Patients die from asphyxia and not exsanguination.
4. Look for cause: most common — pulmonary tuberculosis, lung cancer, bronchiectasis; less common — lung abscess, mycetoma, arterio-venous malformation and pulmonary embolism; rare — coagulopathy, collagen vascular disease (including Wegener's granuloma), Goodpasture's syndrome, and mitral stenosis.

Investigations
1. Blood investigations: FBC, PT/PTT, electrolytes, urea and creatinine, ABG, cross-match.
2. Radiology: CXR — usually a focal abnormality; may be normal if the hemoptysis is from cancer in the central airway, focal bronchiectasis or chronic bronchitis. Diffuse infiltrates bilaterally are seen with pulmonary hemorrhage syndromes. CT scans may help localise the bleeding.

Management
1) Secure airway — large suction device (Yankeur).
2) Supplemental oxygen.
3) Two peripheral IVs (large bore).
4) IV Fluids (Normal saline or gelafundin) if hypotensive and provide blood products as needed.
5) Cough suppressants — phensedryl 15 mls tid.
6) Antibiotics (e.g. second-generation cephalosporin or beta lactam/beta-lactamase inhibitor).

7) Intubation if torrential bleeding or severe hypoxemia — lie patient with bleeding side dependent. Consider a double-lumen endotracheal tube to contain bleeding to one lung.
8) Once airway is secure, bronchoscopy can be attempted to localise the source of bleeding. However, rigid bronchoscopy is the procedure of choice for better suction and ventilation
8) Angiogram to embolise the supplying arteries.
9) Surgical resection if embolisation fails to control the bleeding.

PLEURAL EFFUSION
CHIN NYAT KOOI

Pathophysiology
Fluid collects in the pleural space when secretion of fluid exceeds resorption.

Hydrostatic, oncotic and intrapleural pressures regulate fluid movement in pleural space.

Clinical evaluation
1. Assess respiratory status and hemodynamics.
2. Ask for breathlessness, pleuritic chest pain, cough, hemoptysis, fever, and systemic history for cause.
3. If effusion > 500 mls: diminished chest movement, stony dullness on percussion, absent breath sound.
4. Examine for systemic causes: infection, malignancy, cardiac failure, renal cause, vasculitis.

Investigations
1. Blood investigations: FBC, electrolytes, urea and creatinine, liver function tests, PT, PTT, and specific investigations depending on suspected cause (e.g. vasculitis, malignancy).
2. Imaging: CXR (lateral views and lateral decubitus may be helpful), CT thorax in loculated effusions or complicated effusions.
3. Thoracocentesis* +/– pleural biopsy. Send fluid to biochemistry for glucose, protein, LDH, pH; hematology lab for cytospin (cell count and differential); micro lab for Gram smear and culture, AFB culture; pathology lab for cytology. The pH sample is to be taken anaerobically into an ABG syringe and send in ice.
4. Bronchoscopy if mass suspected or suspected proximal obstruction.
5. Thoracoscopy, or thoracotomy in complicated loculated effusions or empyema.

*Thoracocentesis
1. Explain the procedure and obtain consent.
2. Check for coagulopathy.
3. Approach from back, medial to the angle of scapula, one intercostal space below the upper level of dullness to percussion; seat the patient leaning forward, with arms folded on a bed table.
4. Aseptic technique. Scrub, glove and mask. Clean the skin (methylated spirit and iodine) and drape. Use a 21G or 23G needle for local analgesia with 1% lignocaine, In-filtrate the skin and then proceed down to the pleura. Penetrate the pleural space and confirm effusion is present.
5. Use a 50 mL syringe attached to a 14G or 16G venula and aspirate 30–50 ml of pleural fluid for investigations through the same site.
6. During the diagnostic tap, the operator may decide: to stop after aspirating 50 ml; or proceed to "drain till dry" if the fluid looks clear (not more than 1.5 L at any one time, to avoid re-expansion pulmonary edema); or to insert a chest tube if the fluid is cloudy, frankly purulent or bloody.
7. Observe closely for 24 hrs.
8. CXR to exclude pneumothorax.

Diagnosis
1. Pleural fluid studies:
   (i) biochemistry panel — total protein, LDH, and glu-cose (distinguish between transudate and exudate): transudate — fluid total protein < 3 g/dl; exudate — pleural fluid/serum total protein ratio > 0.5, or pleu-ral fluid/serum LDH ratio > 0.6, or pleural fluid LDH > 2/3 the upper limit of serum LDH; glucose — if < 3.3 mmol/L, suggests infection (bacterial, TB), malignancy, or inflammation (RA, SLE, oesophageal rupture).
   (ii) pH: if < 7.3, has same implication as low glucose; if < 7.1 in a parapneumonic effusion, together with

glucose < 2.2 mmol/L and LDH > 1000 U/L, chest tube drainage is indicated (high-risk effusion).
(iii) cells (cytospin), if predominantly: PMNs — acute exudates (parapneumonic, PE, etc); lymphocytes (esp if > 85%) — TB, lymphoma, sarcoid, other carcinoma.

2. Causes:
   (i) Transudative: congestive cardiac failure, SVC obstruction, constrictive pericarditis, liver cirrhosis with ascites, hypoalbuminemia, nephrotic syndrome, peritoneal dialysis, myxoedema, urinothorax, Meig's syndrome.
   (ii) Exudative: Infections [parapneumonic effusions, empyema (bacterial, TB, fungal, mycoplasma, viral, others), liver/splenic abscess, splenic infarct, oesophageal perforation], malignancies (primary and secondary lung tumours, lymphomas and leukemias, pleural mesothelioma), immunologic (SLE, RA, MCTD, WG, Sjogren's, Dressler syndrome), others (pulmonary embolism, pancreatitis, asbestosis, uremic effusion), lymphatic problems [chylothorax, lymphagiomyomatosis (LAM), Yellow Nail Syndrome], iatrogenic (CVP misplacement, oesophageal sclerotherapy, after abdominal surgery, drug-induced).

Management
1. Oxygen supplement for breathless patients.
2. Treat underlying causes.
3. Therapeutic chest-tube for relief of symptoms (large effusions), high-risk effusions or frank empyema, when frequent or repeated tap is required (e.g. malignant effusion) followed by pleurodesis.

Chest-tube. Aseptic technique. Place the tube in the most dependent portion of the pleural space with free-flowing effusion. The 6th intercostal space in the mid-axillary line is usually chosen for patient comfort. Imaging help required for loculated effusions. Large-bore chest-tube (22Fr–28Fr) is preferred for drainage of pus and blood. Local analgesia. Small skin incision. The tube is inserted by the trocar method ($\pm$ blunt dissection). Once the pleura is punctured, the trocar is withdrawn slightly so that the tip is not protruding; guide the tube posteriorly towards the base. The trocar is removed and the tube connected to an underwater drainage bottle. An anchoring as well as a purse-string suture (2/0 Silk or Prolene) are usually applied to secure the tube. Check the tube position with a PA and lateral CXR. Remove the tube when drainage is < 50 mL/day, and CXR showed clearance of effusion.

4. Treat the underlying cause.
5. **Pleurodesis** for malignant effusion. Pre-med with pethidine 30 minutes before procedure. Clamp the chest tube and disconnect. Clean the nozzle area and adjacent areas with methylated spirit and iodine, then drape. Instill 100 mg of lignocaine in 20 mL of normal saline first through the tube, then reclamped. 10 mins later, the talc slurry (5 g in 100 mL of normal saline per dose) is instilled; the syringe must be gently agitated during instillation so that the talc will remain in suspension. Finally the tube is flushed with 20 ml of normal saline to ensure all the talc is in the pleural cavity and not in the chest-tube. Reconnect the chest tube to the drainage tube, and clamp for 4 hrs. Turning is not required. Additional oral analgesia may be required. The tube can be unclamped at the end of 4 hours, and allowed to drain passively. Repeat a CXR the next day, and the tube can be removed if the CXR showed no increase in effusion and the overnight drainage from the tube is < 100ml.
6. For empyemas, consider use of fibrinolytic agent (streptokinase 250,000 IU in 100 mL NS) to improve drainage, and early referral for thoracotomy in the absence of clearcut clinical improvement to medical therapy.

PNEUMOTHORAX
CHIN NYAT KOOI

Definitions
1. Primary spontaneous pneumothorax: a pneumothorax (ptx) that occurs spontaneously in a person without underlying lung disease; more common in man, most are between 15–40 yrs old; smoking increases the risk, so does a tall, thin (Marfanoid) habitus.
2. Secondary spontaneous pneumothorax: occurring in a person with underlying lung disease (COPD, asthma, bronchiectasis).

Clinical evaluation
1. Assess vitals (respiratory distress or tension pneumo-thorax).
2. History of trauma, foreign body aspiration.
3. Chest pain and dyspnoea are common complaints.
4. Other relevant past medical history.
5. Examine for diminished breath sounds with hyper-resonance on percussion. Look for tracheal shift. Presence of surgical emphysema.

Investigations
1. Blood investigations: ABG as indicated, FBC, electrolytes, urea and creatinine and PT/PTT.
2. CXR (PA) — an expiration film may be required if the pneumothorax is not apparent in the normal CXR in full inspiration. Approximate size of pneumothorax (%) = $100\% - [(d^3/D^3) \times 100\%]$, where D = diameter of the hemithorax at the level of dome of diaphragm, and d = diameter of the collapsed lung.
3. CT thorax may be needed in some ventilated patients — pneumothorax may not apparent on a supine AP film. Look also for pleural blebs (high-resolution).

Management

1. Conservative: pneumothorax < 15% of the hemithorax, and not clinically dyspneic — observe as an outpatient, and review CXR in 1 week (rate of absorption about 1.25% per day); advise to rest at home, not take part in vigorous sports, diving, weight-lifting, and not to travel in unpressurised aircrafts until the pneumothorax has fully resolved.
2. Admit to hospital.
3. Supplemental O_2 accelerates the rate of pleural air absorption by 4 times.
4. Tube thoracostomy (chest-tube insertion) — alternative is simple aspiration. Use chest-tubes of size 20–24G. Insert in the 4th or 5th ICS, mid-axillary line, under LA. An alternative site is the 2nd ICS in the anterior chest wall. Loculated pneumothorax in patients with previous pleural adhesions should be drained under image guidance. Attach the drain to an underwater seal and allow to drain passively. Check the patency of tube daily by observing the fluctuation of the water level with respiration or sniffing. Consider pleurodesis once the tube has stopped bubbling and the CXR shows no pneumothorax. Recurrence more common without pleurodesis (25% to 50% per annum).
5. Pleurodesis (see page 57).
6. Quit smoking.
7. Treat any lung conditions.
8. Thoracoscopy recommended when lungs have not re-expanded after 7 days of drainage despite patent chest tube, recurrent pneumothorax post-pleurodesis, or have blebs or bulla evident on CXR or CT thorax, persistent air-leak, spontaneous hemopneumothorax where blood loss is massive (> 1000 ml/day) or rapid (with hypotension, tachycardia) (urgent referral), high risk occupation such as air-plane pilot or deep sea diver for surgical pleurodesis.
9. Open thoracostomy usually done if thoracoscopy is unavailable or failed.

10. When there is persistent air-leak and patient is not fit for surgery, tube drainage can be continued, or a Heimlich valve may be used. The air-leak usually resolves eventually. Meanwhile vigilant tube site care is recommended to avoid wound infection and empyema formation. Chest physiotherapy and ambulation also help to reduce risk of hypostatic pneumonia.

NON-INVASIVE MECHANICAL VENTILATION AND CPAP

LEE KANG HOE

Mechanical ventilation is traditionally accomplished by the insertion of an endotracheal or nasopharyngeal tube, followed by positive pressure ventilation. Complications can develop from this approach, in addition to the requirement for ICU facilities.

Complications relate to the placement of the tube (aspiration, laryngeal injury, hypotension, hypoxemia, tracheal stenosis) and the increased risk of pulmonary infections.

Non-invasive ventilation includes various techniques of augmenting alveolar ventilation without an endotracheal airway. This allows the therapy to be provided out of ICU. This type of ventilation may take 2 forms: non-invasive (intermittent) positive pressure ventilation (NPPV) — also commonly called BiPAP (but this is a tradename); negative pressure ventilator.

Continuous positive airway pressure (mask CPAP) — this is **not** a ventilation device. This means there is no assistance to ventilation. In CPAP, there is a negative pressure deflection during inspiration, while for NPPV, there is a positive pressure supported inspiratory phase. CPAP is beneficial for certain cases of respiratory failure and will also be discussed below.

Basis for benefit

1. CPAP: In acute respiratory failure, there may be shunts or low V/Q units leading to hypoxemia. Applied PEEP will promote alveolar recruitment and thus increase FRC leading to a decrease in shunt. Furthermore, cardiac output can be augmented by reducing afterload. If patient is intravascularly depleted, there may be a fall in cardiac output instead. For COPD patients, the development of intrinsic PEEP from dynamic hyperinflation (airflow limitation, disadvantaged respiratory muscles) can account

for 43% of the total work of breathing. Counterbalancing iPEEP with applied PEEP will reduce this work as well as reduce the degree of dynamic hyperinflation.
2. NPPV, by providing a positive boost as well during inspiration will aid the fatigued respiratory muscles.

Indications
1. Acute or chronic respiratory failure (type I and type II failure).
2. Acute pulmonary oedema (CPAP preferable).
3. Chronic congestive heart failure with sleep-related breathing disorder (CPAP).

Exclusion criteria:
1. Inability to protect their airway.
2. Failure of prior attempts at noninvasive ventilation.
3. Hemodynamic instability/life-threatening arrhythmias.
4. Impaired mental status.
5. Inability to use nasal or face mask.

How to use the devices
1. CPAP mask — High-flow (turn up the dial to full), and start at FiO_2 of 100% with PEEP 5.0 cm H_2O. Monitor with pulse oximeter and arterial blood gas for $PaCO_2$ measurements. The patient should respond within 15–20 minutes. Consider discontinuation if patient is increasingly drowsy, uncooperative, or feels increased dysponea, with a rising $PaCO_2$. Try to provide rests in between CPAP sessions, e.g. 4 hours on and 30 minutes off. Higher levels of PEEP (7.5 or 10 cm H_2O) can be employed if the patient is still hypoxemic or obese with decreased chest wall compliance. Monitor for hypotension.
2. NPPV (BiPAP) — Nasal masks can be employed initially, with the option of a full face mask if there is significant mouth-breathing. Set iPAP at 10 to 20 cmH_2O, and ePAP at 5 cmH_2O. Supplemental oxygen may be needed, and this is provided directly to the nasal mask as an external

attachment. Monitor as for CPAP. If there is significant mouth-breathing, consider a face-mask. The machine should be on spontaneous/time mode with a back-up rate of 14 to 18 breaths per minute, with inspiratory time at 30%. Alternative NPPV set-up utilises the normal ventilator with a mask, and using the pressure-control mode.

RENAL

COMMON FLUID AND ELECTROLYTE PROBLEMS

TAN CHORH CHUAN

HYPONATRAEMIA

Diagnosis
Serum $[Na^+]$ < 135 mmol/l; usually no symptoms till serum $[Na^+]$ < 125 mmol/l. Symptoms arise from cerebral oedema: apathy, nausea, abnormal sensorium, pseudobulbar palsy and seizures.

Pseudohyponatraemia: Not an issue if direct-reading potentiometry utilised (e.g. NUH). If other methods used, suspect pseudohyponatraemia if severe hyperlipidaemia, hyperproteinaemia (measured plasma osmolality normal), hyperglycaemia or mannitol administration (plasma osmolality high).

Clinical evaluation (determine cause) and investigations
ASSESS PATIENT'S VOLUME STATUS: history of fluid loss, fluid balance on input-output chart, postural hypotension, skin turgor, mucosa, JVP and neck veins.

Check serum osmolality (normal 275–300 mOsm/kg), and spot urine osmolality and $[Na^+]$.

1. Patient clinically volume depleted: urine $[Na^+]$ < 10 mmol/l (non-renal losses) — gastrointestinal loss, third space loss e.g. peritonitis, burns; urine $[Na^+]$ > 20 mmol/l (renal losses) — diuretic (mainly thiazides), osmotic diuresis eg severe hyperglycaemia, salt losing nephritis with renal impairment, adrenal insufficiency (usually also hyperkalaemia). Hyponatraemia is due to appropriate ADH release from hypovolaemia. Thus, urine osmolality appropriately increased (>100 mOsm/kg).
2. Hypervolaemic: cardiac failure, cirrhosis, nephrotic syndrome, advanced renal failure.

3. Euvolaemic: glucocorticoid deficiency and hypothyroidism; drugs e.g. chlopropamide, tolbutamide, cyclophosphamide, vincristine, carbamazepine, amitriptyline, haloperidol (some of these act by causing SIADH); Syndrome of inappropriate ADH secretion (SIADH) — urine osmolality inappropriately high (> 100 mOsm/kg) for serum osmolality (< 275 mosm/kg); urine [Na^+] >40 mmol/l, more common causes include brain infections/tumours, cerebrovascular accident, post-surgery, pneumonia, small cell lung cancer, drugs.

Note: Hyponatraemia may be due to more than one cause, e.g. underlying SIADH with volume depletion from vomiting. Serial evaluation will clarify diagnosis.

Acute management
1. Treat underlying cause of hyponatraemia: volume depleted patient — give IV 0.9% NaCl till clinically volume replete and, treat underlying cause for extracellular fluid depletion; hypervolaemic patient — treat cardiac failure; stop possible culpable medications.
2. Restrict fluid intake to 500 ml/day in hypervolaemic or euvolaemic patients.
3. Asymptomatic patients with no reversible cause for hyponatraemia (e.g. cirrhosis) and serum [Na^+] > 130 mmol/l — leave alone but monitor serum [Na^+].
4. If acute hyponatraemia and neurological symptoms, raise serum [Na^+] with 3% NaCl to 120 mmol/l or until symptoms improve. If serum Na^+ < 120 mmol/l without symptoms, similarly correct to 120 mmol/l. Thereafter, correct hyponatraemia slowly.

Estimate Na^+ replacement as follows:
Na^+ deficit = 0.6 × Body weight × (desired plasma [Na^+] − current plasma [Na^+])

Example, to raise serum [Na^+] from 108 to 120 mmol/l in symptomatic 50 kg patient,
Na^+ deficit = 0.6 × 50 × (120−108) = 360 mmol

Since 1 litre of 3% NaCl contains 513 mmol Na⁺, patient needs 700 ml of 3% NaCl.

To correct deficit over 24 hours, give 3% NaCl at 30 ml/hour (700ml ÷ 24 hours). Infuse at 50–75 ml/hour for first 3–4 hours because of presence of symptoms.

5. If patient at risk of pulmonary oedema from saline infusion OR if urine osmolality > 400 mOsm/kg in SIADH, give frusemide (e.g. 40 mg IV tds) to increase urinary free water excretion.
6. Monitor serum [Na⁺] closely particularly in first 48 hours.
7. DO NOT correct serum [Na⁺] faster than 12 mmol/l per day and AVOID correction to > 135 mol/l. Over-rapid correction can cause neurological deterioration, central pontine myelinolysis and death.
8. For chronic SIADH — fluid 500 ml/day, oral frusemide 20–40 mg bd with KCl 0.6–1.2 g om and oral NaCl 2 tabs tds (to prevent hypovolaemia; 1 tab = 300mg = 5 mmol Na⁺).

HYPERNATRAEMIA

Diagnosis
Serum [Na⁺] > 150 mmol/l. Symptoms from lethargy, tremulousness to spasticity, fits and coma. Thirst usually prevents hypernatraemia, which develops only when hypotonic fluid losses occur together with disturbed water intake, e.g. ill patient unable to drink.

Clinical evaluation (determine cause) and investigations
CRITICAL TO ASSESS PATIENT'S VOLUME STATUS.
Check serum osmolality, spot urine osmolality and [Na⁺] as indicated below.

1. Volume depleted (Na⁺ and water loss but water loss greater): urine [Na⁺] < 10 mmol/l unless renal disease present, urine osmolality high (non-renal loss) —

osmotic diarrhoea (e.g. lactulose, some gastroenteritides), burns, sweating; urine $[Na^+] > 20$ mmol/l (renal loss) — osmotic diuresis (mannitol, uncontrolled diabetes mellitus, post-obstructive diuresis), intrinsic renal disease.

2. Hypervolaemic (least common): excessive administration of hypertonic $NaHCO_3$ or 3% NaCl, sea-water drowning.

3. Euvolaemic i.e. primarily water loss (commonest): insensible water loss in patients unable to drink (e.g. comatose state); central diabetes insipidus (idiopathic, head injury, brain tumours and infections, posthypophysectomy) and thirst centre also affected or no access to water; nephrogenic diabetes insipidus (chronic renal diseases, drugs e.g. lithium and amphotericin B, chronic hypercalcaemia) with inadequate water intake.

Acute management
1. In volume-depleted patient, with circulatory manifestations (eg orthostatic hypotension), give 0.9% or 0.45% NaCl till haemodynamically stable. Subsequently, correct hypernatraemia with IV 0.45% NaCl (if need to replace continuing Na^+ loss) or 5% dextrose. Water should also be given orally.

2. In hypervolaemic patient, stop excess Na^+ administration and give diuretics (e.g. IV frusemide) to excrete excess Na^+. Correct hypernatraemia with water orally and/or with IV 5%.

3. In euvolaemic patient, correct with water orally and/or with IV 5% dextrose as follows:

Example, to estimate water volume required to reduce serum $[Na^+]$ from 154 to 140 mmol/l in a 75 kg man:

Total body water = $0.6 \times$ body weight = 0.6×75 kg
= 45 litres

Total body water for serum $[Na^+]$ to be 140 mmol/l = $(154 \div 140) \times 45$ = 49.5 litres

Water volume needed to reduce serum [Na⁺] to 140
mmol/l = 49.5 − 45 = 4.5 litres
To correct over 48 hours with IV 5% dextrose, give at
100 ml/hour + additional 40 ml/hour (for insensible water
loss).

4. In central diabetes insipidus (most commonly in severe
   head-injured patients), DDAVP can be given (IV 2–4 µg
   bd, dose adjusted to urine output and osmolality).
5. Serum [Na⁺] must be monitored closely particularly in
   first 48 hours.
6. Treat underlying cause of hypernatraemia.
7. Hypernatraemia should be corrected at a rate not
   > 12 mmol/l/day. Over-rapid correction can cause cerebral oedema, fits, permanent neurological deficits and
   death.

HYPOKALAEMIA

Diagnosis
Serum $[K^+] < 3.5$ mmol/l; marked symptoms uncommon till
serum $[K^+] < 2.5$–3.0 mmol/l. Hypokalaemia can induce
cardiac arrhythmias especially if underlying heart disease or
digoxin treatment. Other symptoms: muscle weakness, ileus,
rhabdomyolysis; impaired urinary concentrating ability and
renal tubulointerstitial damage with chronic hypokalaemia.

Clinical evaluation (determine cause) and investigations
Cause usually obvious clinically. In difficult cases, measure
24–hour urine K^+ or fractional K^+ excretion (FE_K) = (Spot
urine $[K^+] \div$ Plasma $[K^+]) \times$ (Plasma[Cr] µmol/l $\div$ Spot urine
[Cr] µmol/L)

1. Inadequate intake: K^+-free IV fluids in patient on 'Nil-by-
   mouth"; low dietary intake (rare). Urine $[K^+] < 25$ mmol/
   24 hours.

2. K+ deficit from increased losses: urine [K+] < 20 mmol/
   24 hours, FE_K < 0.06 (non-renal loss) — diarrhoea/laxa-
   tive abuse (associated normal-anion gap metabolic acidosis); urine K+ > 20 mmol/24 hours, FE_K > 0.06 (renal
   loss) — loop and thiazide diuretics, with hypertension
   (malignant hypertension, renal artery stenosis, Conn's
   syndrome), renal tubular acidosis (normal-anion gap
   acidosis), Mg^{++} depletion, amphotericin (up to 50%
   patients), Bartter's syndrome (rare), vomiting or nasogastric suction (associated metabolic alkalosis).
3. K+ redistribution from extracellular to intracellular fluid:
   metabolic or respiratory alkalosis, insulin excess (e.g.
   treatment of uncontrolled diabetes) or acute glucose load,
   β-adrenergic agonists (nebulised salbutamol), periodic
   paralysis.
4. Hypokalaemia in dialysis patients: CAPD patients lose K+
   in the dialysate; HD patients — hypokalaemia on immediate "post-dialysis" samples is usually because equili-
   bration has not yet occured. If serum [K+] > 3 mmol/l,
   leave alone. For lower values or if in doubt, repeat serum
   [K+]. INAPPROPRIATE K+ REPLACEMENT CAN CAUSE
   SEVERE HYPERKALAEMIA.

Acute management

1. Serum [K+] of 2.5–3.5 mmol/l, with no significant heart
   disease or concurrent digoxin treatment, treat underlying
   disorder (e.g. diarrhoea) and replace K+ orally (e.g. SpanK
   1.2 g tds [= 48 mmol/day] or mist KCl 10–20 ml tds
   (1 mmol K+ per ml). If patient on "Nil-by-mouth", give
   IV KCl 60–80 mmol/day in divided doses (KCl concentration in IV fluid should not be > 60 mmol/l). Omit or
   reduce K+ replacement in patients with severe renal failure or dialysis.
2. If symptomatic (e.g. muscular weakness) or serum
   [K+] < 2.5 mmol/l, do ECG stat. Replace K+ orally (mist
   KCl 20 ml 6 hourly) and by IV infusion, e.g. 20 mmol
   KCl in 100–200 ml 0.9% NaCl over 2 hours, then repeat
   same dose over 2 hours, then check serum [K+] stat.

Repeat cycle until symptoms and ECG changes improve, and/or serum [K+] > 3 mmol/l, after which replace with oral KCl alone.

3. Maximum IV replacement rate is 20 mmol/hour. Avoid dextrose-containing fluids.
4. Order K+ in small amounts at a time, e.g. 20 mmol over 2 hours twice, rather than 40 mmol over 4 hours, to avoid accidental over-rapid administration of large amount of K+.
5. Give through large peripheral veins.
6. Beware "rebound hyperkalaemia" when treating hypo-kalaemia due to redistribution of K+ (e.g. thyrotoxic periodic paralysis).
7. In CAPD patients with severe hypokalaemia, give oral replacement and intraperitoneal KCl 12 mmol/2 litres dialysate for each PD exchange till serum [K+] > 3 mmol/l.
8. Treat underlying cause of hypokalaemia.

HYPERKALAEMIA

Diagnosis
Serum [K+] > 5.0 mmol/l. Haemolysis of blood specimen or use of a tight tourniquet around an exercising arm (e.g. opening and closing hand), can result in "pseudohyperkalaemia".

HYPERKALAEMIA CAN INDUCE CARDIAC ARRHYTHMIAS, VENTRICULAR FIBRILLATION AND DEATH.

ECG changes related to serum [K+]:

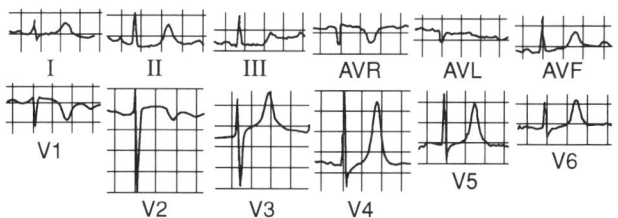

Clinical evaluation (determine cause) and investigations

1. ECG must be done if serum $[K^+] > 6.0$ mmol/l.
2. Hyperkalaemia must be considered in differential diagnosis of all broad-complex tachycardias.
3. Increased intake or administration of K^+ — mainly in patients with impaired renal K^+ excretion e.g. renal failure, hypoaldosteronism.
4. Decreased renal excretion: renal failure — reduced ability to excrete acute K^+ load, therefore increased K^+ intake or endogenous release (e.g. rhabdomyolysis); spironolactone, ACE-inhibitors; chronic renal failure by itself does not usually cause hyperkalaemia until CCT < 10 ml/min.
5. Hypoaldosteronism: hyporeninaemic hypoaldosteronism — most have mild-to-moderate renal impairment, 50% have diabetes mellitus, NSAIDs, ACE-inhibitors, spironolactone are reversible causes; primary adrenal insufficiency.
6. K^+ redistribution from intracellular to extracellular fluid: metabolic acidosis; insulin deficiency and hyperglycaemia (uncontrolled diabetes, hyperglycaemia in dialysis patients); hypercatabolic state (rhabdomyolysis, trauma, severe sepsis, tumour lysis).

Acute management

1. Stop all K^+ supplements and K^+-sparing diuretics (e.g. spironolactone). Low K^+-diet.
2. Serum $[K^+] < 6.5$ mmol/l, no significant cardiac disease and no ECG changes other than peaked T-waves — give oral resonium 15 g tds $\pm$ IV 10 U soluble insulin with 40 ml of 50% dextrose.
3. Serum $[K^+] > 6.5$ mmol/l, or any level of hyperkalaemia with ECG changes other than peaked T-waves present:
   - continuous ECG monitoring
   - IV 10 ml 10% calcium gluconate over 3–5 minutes
   - IV 10 U soluble insulin with 40 ml of 50% dextrose
   - Nebulised salbutamol 10 mg in 2 ml normal saline
   - Resonium 15 g stat and 4–8 hourly OR Resonium enema 30 g stat and 4–8 hourly

- IV 4.2% $NaHCO_3$ 50–100 ml over 30 min if arterial pH < 7.2
- IV frusemide 40 mg stat if renal function normal or mildly impaired
- If severe renal failure or dialysis patients, urgent dialysis required.

4. Serum $[K^+]$ can rise very quickly in hypercatabolic states eg crush injury, severe sepsis. For these, serum $[K^+]$ must be monitored closely and aggressive treatment instituted at lower levels of hyperkalaemia than outlined above.

5. Treat underlying cause of hyperkalaemia.

6. Serum $[K^+]$ must be closely monitored after treatment.

METABOLIC ACIDOSIS

Diagnosis

Arterial pH < 7.36 due to a primary decrease in plasma $[HCO_{3-}]$. Plasma $[HCO_{3-}]$ is measured as total venous serum $[CO_2]$. In *pure* metabolic acidosis, arterial pCO_2 is reduced by $1–1.5 \times$ decrease in venous $[CO_2]$. Severe acidosis causes depressed myocardial contractility and response to inotropes, hypotension, and altered conscious state.

Establish the cause of metabolic acidosis

1. Calculate serum anion gap from Renal panel: $([Na^+] + [K^+]) - ([Cl^-] + [CO_2])$
   (i) Normal anion gap (12–20 mmol/l): Diarrhoea, acetazolamide use, renal tubular acidosis,
   (ii) High anion gap (> 20 mmol/l): Diabetic ketoacidosis; Lactic acidosis, e.g. from shock, severe sepsis, liver failure; Salicylate poisoning; Methanol and ethylene glycol intoxication — suspect if measured serum osmolality is 15–20 mOsm/kg > calculated serum osmolality ($2[Na^+] + [Glucose] + [Urea]$); Renal failure.

Acute management
1. Treat underlying cause.
2. If severe acidosis (arterial pH < 7.2), give IV 8.4% $NaHCO_3$ 50–100 ml over 1–2 hours, then recheck arterial pH. Do not correct pH to > 7.25 with IV Na HCO_3. Monitor serum $[K^+]$.
3. If severe acidosis in patient with severe fluid overload, consider dialysis.
4. For chronic acidosis, give oral Na HCO_3 0.5–2 g/day (12 mmol HCO_3 per g) OR sodium citrate (Shohl's solution) 10–60 ml/day (1 mmol of salt per ml).

METABOLIC ALKALOSIS

Diagnosis
Arterial pH > 7.45 due to a primary increase in plasma $[HCO_{3-}]$; arterial pCO_2 increased by $0.25 - 1 \times$ rise in venous $[CO_2]$ in pure metabolic alkalosis. Symptoms not specific, may relate to volume depletion or hypokalaemia.

Establish the cause of metabolic alkalosis
Cause can almost always be identified from the history. Evaluation of the patient's volume status is critical. Check spot urine $[Cl^-]$.
1. Patient **volume depleted** — (spot urine $[Cl^-]$ < 20 mmol/l; NaCl-reponsive alkalosis): vomiting/nasogastric suction (common); diuretics (common); rapid correction of chronic hypercapnia (e.g. by mechanical ventilation) in volume depleted patient
2. Patient **not volume depleted** (spot urine $[Cl^-]$ > 20 mmol/l):
   (i) Primary hyperaldosteronism: associated hypertension with hypokalaemia,
   (ii) Excessive alkali administration (e.g. Na HCO_3, antacids) especially in renal failure,
   (iii) Massive blood transfusion (> 10 units blood containing citrate as anticoagulant),
   (iv) High-dose penicillin treatment.

Management
1. Treat underlying cause. In patients with continuing loss of gastric secretions (e.g. nasogastric suction), give ranitidine or omeprazole to reduce gastric HCl loss.
2. For NaCl-responsive forms of metabolic alkalosis, give IV 0.9% NaCl to correct volume depletion. Monitor response by serial [Cl⁻] which remains < 25 mmol/l till Cl⁻ deficit corrected. Correct associated hypokalaemia with KCl replacement.
3. For alkalosis due to primary hyperaldosteronism, give spironolactone 50 mg tds orally. Correct associated hypokalaemia.
4. For patients with metabolic alkalosis and hypervolaemia, e.g. cardiac failure, consider acetazolamide (250 mg om-bd; caution/avoid in renal failure, chronic hypercapnia) with potassium supplementation.

ACUTE RENAL FAILURE
LEONG SEE ODD

Clinical evaluation

1. Recognise presence of renal failure: may have uremic symptoms, raised serum urea and creatinine ± hyperkalaemia and acidosis. Oliguria (urine output < 20 ml/hour) may be present but is not essential for diagnosis.

2. Determine if renal failure is acute, chronic (features of chronicity — past history of renal disease or urine abnormalities, raised serum creatinine in previous admission, sallow appearance, oedema or uraemic symptoms in preceding months, small kidneys on ultrasound) or acute-on-chronic.

3. Identify acute, reversible causes for renal failure.

4. Pre-renal causes — reduced glomerular filtration rate resulting from a decrease in renal perfusion pressure or intense renal vasoconstriction, or both.

   (i)   volume depletion secondary to: excessive diuresis, haemorrhage, gastrointestinal fluid losses, third space loss, e.g. burns.

   (ii) cardiac and vascular causes: AMI, CCF, renal artery stenosis.

   (iii) peripheral vasodilatation: G-negative sepsis, anti-hypertensive drugs.

   (iv) increased renal vascular resistance: hepatorenal syndrome, drugs (NSAIDs, cyclosporine).

4. Pre-renal azotemia precedes and predisposes to ATN, in which renal structural damage is present. Evaluation of the intravascular volume status is crucial: History of blood or fluid loss, change in body weight, postural hypotension, skin turgor; mucous membrane moisture. Early recognition and vigorous treatment can restore renal function. Delays in treatment can result in prolonged period of renal impairment.

6. Post-renal causes (obstruction to flow of urine):

   (i)   urethral obstruction: valves, strictures.

    (ii)   bladder neck obstruction: prostatic hypertrophy or carcinoma, autonomic neuropathy and ganglionic blocking agent.

    (iii)   ureteral obstruction (bilateral to cause ARF): intra-ureteral (stones, clots, sloughed papillae), extra-ureteral (pelvic and bladder carcinoma, retroperi-toneal fibrosis).

    Rapid relief of obstruction is critical.

7. Intrinsic renal diseases:

    (i)   primary renal, systemic and vascular diseases: rapidly progressive glomerulonephritis, acute post-streptococcal glomerulonephritis, SLE, vasculitides, Goodpasture's syndrome, rhabdomyolysis.

    (ii)   acute interstitial nephritis: antibiotic-induced (penicillins, cephalosporins, sulphonamides), miscs (allopurinol, NSAIDs), infections e.g. leptospirosis.

    (iii)   nephrotoxins: anti-infectives (aminoglycosides, vancomycin, amphotericin), cytotoxic agents (cisplatin), iodine containing radio-contrast media, heavy metals (mercury), organic solvents.

8. Diagnosis usually obvious clinically. Renal biopsy may be necessary if cause of ARF not apparently clinically. Treatment is directed at underlying conditions and cessation of insults to kidney. Dialysis may be needed to tide over acute events. Recovery depends on underlying condition.

Investigations

1. Blood: FBC, electrolytes, urea and creatinine, calcium, phosphate, ABG, other tests as indicated (e.g. ANA, ANCA, etc.)

2. Imaging: CXR, AXR (if indicated), ultrasound kidneys for size and to exclude obstruction.

3. ECG.

4. On urine microscopy, presence of abundant red cells, red and white cells casts, heavy proteinuria (>3 g/24 hours) usually suggestive of acute glomerulonephritis.

5. Urinary diagnostic indices.

Index	pre-renal ARF	Acute tubular necrosis
urine sodium (mmol/l)	< 20	> 40
urine osmolarity (mosmol/l)	> 500	< 350
urine/plasma urea	> 8	< 3
urine/plasma creatinine	> 40	< 20
fractional Na excretion $(U_{Na}/P_{Na} \times P_{Cr}/U_{Cr})$	< 1	> 2

Management

1. Identify and vigorously correct acute reversible factors contributing to renal failure.
2. Treat complications of ARF:
   (i) If fluid overload present — give IV frusemide 40–160 mg stat and 6–8 hourly.
   (ii) If hyperkalaemia present, treat as described in section on electrolyte abnormalities,
   (iii) If severe metabolic acidosis present (pH < 7.2) treat as described.
3. Consult Renal Physician-on-call for possible dialysis if severe complications of ARF are present, if patient has disturbed sensorium due to ARF, or if the patient is in a hypercatabolic state (e.g. multiple trauma, severe sepsis, rhabdomyolysis)
4. Look actively for sepsis and treat with IV antibiotics if there is any suspicion of infection.

ACUTE PROBLEMS COMMONLY ENCOUNTERED IN DIALYSIS PATIENTS
EVAN LEE

A. Fluid overload
Breathlessness, orthopnoea, raised JVP, lung crackles, pulmonary oedema, peripheral oedema.

Clinical evaluation
1. Commonest cause — missed haemodialysis sessions or PD exchanges, often associated with excessive fluid intake.
2. Acute myocardial infarction or ischaemia; dilated cardiomyopathy.
3. Inappropriate IV fluid therapy including blood transfusion.

Investigations
1. Blood investigations: FBC, electrolytes, urea and creatinine, ABG, CK, CKMB.
2. ECG.
3. CXR.

Management
1. High flow oxygen (intranasal O_2 5 L/min or Ventimask 50%) — monitor pulse oximetry if available (ABG otherwise if patient ill).
2. Contact Renal Physician on call for urgent dialysis.
3. If significant delay till dialysis, give IV frusemide 120 mg or IV bumetanide 5 mg.
4. If patient in respiratory distress from pulmonary oedema, CPAP mask may be considered. If despite 100% oxygen or significant hypercapnia with exhaustion, intubate and ventilate while preparing for dialysis.
5. Treat underlying cause if possible.
6. Patients frequently have associated hyperkalaemia — this should be looked for and treated medically if dialysis cannot be initiated in 1–2 hours.

B . Fever in a patient with a temporary haemodialysis catheter

Double lumen venous dialysis catheters are inserted in the internal jugular, subclavian or femoral vein as temporary access for haemodialysis. In a patient with high fever without an obvious focus of infection, the catheter is the most likely source of infection.

1. Do blood cultures 2 times, FBC, electrolytes, urea and creatinine, and CXR.
2. Give IV cloxacillin 500 mg stat and 6 hourly (or Vancomycin 500 mg to 1 G stat, if MRSA suspected), and IV cefuroxime 750 mg stat and 8 hourly.
3. Consult the Renal Physician-on-call about removal of the dialysis catheter.

C. Peritonitis in a patient on CAPD

Cloudy PD effluent is the commonest and earliest sign. Also abdominal pain, diarrhoea, vomiting, fever.

Management
1. PD fluid taken for cell count and culture at Renal Centre.
2. Order intraperitoneal Vancomycin 1G and Gentamicin 40 mg stat. If the patient had received gentamicin in the preceding 2 months, substitute with intraperitoneal ceftazidime 1 G stat.
3. If patient is diabetic, monitor blood sugar by meter 4 times per day and give SC insulin accordingly.
4. As peritonitis is associated with decreased ultrafiltration, look for signs of fluid overload. If present, the patient may require additional PD exchanges to increase fluid removal.

D. Common electrolyte abnormalities in dialysis patients

1. Hypokalaemia:
   (i) Check when blood test was done with respect to haemodialysis. If test was done immediately post-dialysis, repeat serum K^+ but do not give KCl.
   (ii) In CAPD patients, if serum K^+ between 2.5–3.5 mmol/l, give mist KCl 20 ml tds for 2 days then oral Span K 1.2 g om. If serum K^+ < 2.5 mmol/l, also order intra-peritoneal KCl 12 ml/2 litre bag of dialysate in addition to oral replacement. If serum K < 2.0 mmol/l, give IV KCl 20 mmol in 100 ml Normal saline over 4 hours in addition to oral and IP KCl. Check serum K^+ after IV replacement and at least once daily till stabilised.

2. Hypercalcaemia: This is most often iatrogenic. Stop $CaCO_3$ and calcitriol or 1 α-calcidol.

3. Hyperphosphataemia: If serum phosphate elevated and calcium (mmol/l)-phosphate (mmol/l) product < 6, give oral $CaCO_3$ 625–1250 mg tds with meals as phosphate binder. If calcium-phosphate product > 6, stop $CaCO_3$ and give $Al(OH_3)$ 10–20 ml tds or Alutabs 2 tab tds with meals. Refer to dietician for low-phosphate diet.

E. General considerations in dialysis or ESRF patients

1. In any patient who may require long term dialysis, do not take blood or set heparin plugs in the left upper limb.
2. Do not attempt to take blood from or give drugs or fluids through haemodialysis catheters or AV fistulae.
3. In ESRF patients who have prolonged bleeding from the site of Tenckhoff or the double lumen catheter insertion site, apply direct digital pressure to the area for 10 min, and check BP and pulse rate. If bleeding persists, inform your Resident or Registrar or the Renal Physician-on-call.

NEUROLOGY

CEREBROVASCULAR EMERGENCIES
BENJAMIN ONG and RICHARD CHAN

Stroke is a clinical syndrome characterised by sudden (or subacute) onset of neurological deficit due to disturbances in the cerebral circulation.

Clinical evaluation
1. Diagnosis: suspect a stroke in the following situations:
   (i) Acute focal cerebral dysfunction, e.g. unilateral weakness, unilateral sensory loss, dysphasia, visual disturbances (blindness, visual field cut, diplopia), vertigo, dysarthria.
   (ii) Signs of raised intracranial pressure (ICP) — drowsiness, pupillary changes.
   (iii) Headache, particularly in subarachnoid hemorrhage with accompanying neck stiffness. Headache is also common in intracerebral hemorrhage.
   (iv) Unexplained alteration of consciousness/confusion.
   (v) Seizures.
2. Important to exclude: hypogylcemia, metabolic and toxic (including drugs) encephalopathies, head injury, post-ictal state or seizure.
3. Assess the vital signs.
4. Check for airway protection (gag reflex).
5. Make a diagnosis (usually requires CT head scan) — Is the stroke a cerebral infarction, intracerebral hemorrhage or subarachnoid hemorrhage?

Investigations
1. Blood investigations — FBC, PT/PTT, electrolyes (include hypocount), urea and creatinine.
2. ECG.
3. Radiological — CXR, CT head scan, occasionally MRI.
4. LP for suspected SAH, if CT head is normal.
5. Echocardiography.
6. Carotid artery ultrasound.
7. Angiography as indicated.

Management

1. Resuscitation:

   (i) Airway management — oropharyngeal airway, frequent suctioning, recovery position, nil by mouth, may require intubation followed by tracheostomy.

   (ii) Blood pressure — Excessively high and excessively low blood pressure may cause further neurological deterioration. Maintain blood pressure in the 150–180/80–100 mmHg range. If the blood pressure is high, lower the blood pressure gradually by using nitroglycerin paste, nitroglycerin patch, oral nifepine 10 mg, or IV labetalol 10–20 mg slow bolus. In cases of malignant hypertension, intravenous infusion of nitroprusside may be required. Do not use agents that drop the blood pressure precipitously (e.g. sublingual nifedipine).

2. Supportive measures:

   (i)   Assume all stroke patients to be at risk of aspiration until the swallowing assessment is carried out. Keep the patient "nil by mouth", maintain hydration with an intravenous infusion of normal saline.

   (ii) Maintain blood pressure within the acceptable range, as mentioned above.

   (iii) Keep the blood glucose level within acceptable range (4–10 mmol/L). Use insulin sliding scale to achieve the desirable blood glucose level.

   (iv) If the patient is incontinent, diaper pad is preferable to in-dwelling urinary catheter. In man, condom catheter can also be used.

   (v)   Prescribe anti-embolic stocking and/or subcutaneous heparin (5000 U BID) or Fraxiparine (0.3 ml om.) to prevent deep vein thrombosis in non-ambulant patients.

   (vi) Early assessment by the physical therapist, occupational therapist and speech pathologist. Rehabilitation program should start as soon as the patient is medically stable. Nursing care — prevent bed sores.

(vii) Seizures: If status epilepticus or second observed fir, load with intravenous phenytoin 15 to 20 mg/kg infusion Alternatives include intravenous valproate (600 mg over 30 minutes).

(viii) The development of raised ICP (decreased conscious level, third nerve palsy, periodic respiration) is a bad prognosis, and the patient seldom survives. Hyperventilation, mannitol, and dexamathesone have a limited role as evidence for long-term outcome benefits are lacking.

3. Specific interventions:

(i) The patient has cerebral infarction. Is the patient a candidate for thrombolytic therapy? A neurologist's review is required. The minimum criteria are: treatment can be started < 3 hrs of stroke onset, measurable neurological deficit, infarction is not too large, no contraindication to thrombolysis, and good premorbid functional level. If the patient is not a thrombolytic candidate, prescribe appropriate antiplatelet agents (aspirin 300 mg or ticlopidine 250 mg om or bid) or anticoagulant (heparin — keep PTT 70 to 90 secs, fraxiparine — 0.4 to 0.6 ml bid sc, or warfarin) for progressive infarcts or posterior circulation strokes.

(ii) The patient has an intracerebral hemorrhage. The patient should be rested. Blood pressure management is especially important to reduce the risk of recurrent bleed. Discontinue all anticoagulant or antiplatelet agents.

(iii) The patient has subarachnoid hemorrhage. Strict rest in bed, withhead of bed elevated at 30°. Prescribe analgesics at a sufficiently high dose, e.g., IM codeine phosphate 0.5–1.0 mg/kg 4 to 6 hourly. Keep the patient well hydrated. If there are no contraindications to hyper-hydration, give IV normal saline 3000 ml daily. Start IV nimodipine at 1 mg/hr. If systolic BP is not < 150 mmHg after 3 hours, increase the dose to 2 mg/hr. (Nimodipine should be given for 3 weeks. Oral preparation dose is 60 mg 4 hourly.)

Arrange for cerebral angiography. Consult a neurosurgeon. An interventional radiologist or radiotherapy physician may be consulted if the underlying cause is an arteriovenous malformation.

CNS INFECTIONS
LEE KANG HOE and BENJAMIN ONG

Presents as either:

1) **acute meningitis syndrome** — rapid onset (< 24-48 hours) of fever, headache and/or meningismus, impairment of higher functions. Commonly from pyogenic meningitis (penumococcal, meningococcal, Heamophilus); uncommonly viral encephalitis, subarachnoid bleed, ruptures brain tumour; and rarely viral meningitis, granulomatous meningitis (cryptococcal, mycobacterial), carcinomatous meningitis, and brain tumour.

2) **subacute** — (> 24–48 hours) onset, with gradual or no impairment of higher functions. Commonly due to viral meningitis, viral encephalitis, pyogenic meningitis; uncommonly brain abscess, brain tumour, granulomatous meningitis; rarely CVA and carcinomatous meningitis.

In AIDS, consider toxoplasmosis, cryptococcus, lymphoma, and progressive multifocal leukoencephalopathy.

Investigations
1. Blood: FBC, electrolytes, urea and creatinine, ABG, PT and PTT, Group and save.
2. Imaging: CXR and CT head scan.
3. Septic workup: LP (measure pressure, and CSF for glucose, protein, chloride, cell-count with differential count, gram-stain, cultures, AFB smear and TB culture, Indian ink, antigens, fungal smear and cultures as indicated, viral cultures as indicated), serologies, blood cultures, sputum and urine cultures.

Clinical evaluation
1. CNS infections are considered a *medical emergency* especially those presenting with an acute meningitis syndrome.
2. Rapid history and physical.

3. Assess vital signs, especially airway protection in obtunded patients.
4. Exclude focal neurologic signs or papilloedema.
5. Establish risk factors (include immunosuppression, neurosurgical intervention, trauma).

Management
1. Antibiotics should be administered within **30 minutes**.
2. Once IV plug is set, give antibiotic immediately (Ceftriaxone 2G stat) — this should be given within 30 minutes. Continue with Ceftriaxone 2G q12h for 7 to 10 days. Consider adding on amikacin (500 mg) if there is evidence of CSF leak or invasion. Chloramphenicol if allergy to penicillins. Antibiotics may be altered later as indicated by cultures.
3. Perform LP — if focal neurology or papilloedema, obtain CT head first. Bacterial meningitis (CSF result) — WBC > 1000/mm^3 (mainly polymorphs), glucose reduced, protein > 1 g/L.
4. If viral encephalitis is suspected, give iv acyclovir (10 mg/kg q8h for 14 days) for presumptive herpes simplex encephalitis (mainly affects temporal lobe — obtain EEG, ± MRI).
5. Head chart, and hourly vital signs.
6. If in coma, check for gag — consider airway protection if absent.
7. Treat seizures with phenytoin (15 to 20 mg/kg load with ECG monitoring preferable over 30 minutes).
8. Steroids: indicated for children with H. Influenzae meningitis (dexamethasone 0.15 mg/kg q6h for 4 days), but unclear benefits in adults (may consider in those with positive Gram-stain on CSF and evidence of raised ICP).
9. TB meningitis — treat with standard triple regimen (isoniazid, rifampicin, and pyrazinamide). Add prednisolone 1 mg/kg if neurological signs are present to reduce the likelihood for hydrocephalus.

STATUS EPILEPTICUS
BENJAMIN ONG and RICHARD CHAN

Status epilepticus is a condition in which there is continuous seizure activity. Continuous focal seizure are alarming but seldom life threatening. Continuous generalised seizure, on the other hand, can lead to severe cerebral injury, metabolic derangement and death. Status epilepticus is a medical emergency.

Traditionally, status epilepticus is defined as continuous or near-continuous generalised seizures, without restoration of consciousness between seizures, lasting more than 30 minutes. If institution of therapy is started after 30 minutes of seizures, severe and possibly permanent damage would be developed. For practical purpose, treatment of status epilepticus should be started when the seizure activity has been on-going for 10 minutes.

Clinical evaluation
1. Assess vital signs and temperature.
2. Exclude focal neurological signs or head injury.
3. Look for signs of sepsis.
4. Ask for the following: withdrawal of anticonvulsant in a known epileptic; alcohol withdrawal; drug intoxication or withdrawal; encephalitis; traumatic brain injury; anoxic brain injury, including stroke.

Investigations
1. FBC, electrolyte (include glucose), calcium, phosphate, magnesium, urea and creatinine, liver function tests, toxicology, toxicology screen, drug levels for anti-epileptic drugs.
2. CXR if aspiration concern.
3. CT head as indicated.
4. EEG as indicated.
5. LP if meningitis or encephalitis suspected.
6. Septic workup if indicated.

Management

General measures
1. Give oxygen 24–50% by mask.
2. Turn the patient to the side to prevent aspiration of oral secretion or vomitus. Do not attempt to insert oral airway, intubate or clear oral content while the patient is still seizing.
3. Set up an intravenous line. Give IV thiamine 10 mg immediately, followed by an infusion of glucose 5% solution. If the patient is hypoglycemic, give a bolus injection of 10–50 ml of 50% glucose solution. (Beware of extravasation!)
4. Consider intubation if airway is compromised (absent gag).
5. Monitor the heart rate and blood pressure every five to ten minutes throughout the treatment period.
6. Do not leave the patient until the seizure is controlled.
7. Treat underlying cause.

Abortive therapy
8. Short acting benzodiazepine such as diazepam or lorazepam are useful in aborting seizures. They must be given intravenously. Diazepam can also be given rectally if the foam preparation is available. The dosages are:
    (i) Diazepam: IV or PR 10 mg bolus (maximum dose 20 mg)
    (ii) Lorazepam: IV 2 mg in 2 ml water bolus (maximum dose 4 mg)
9. If the patient continues to seize, consider IV chlormethiazole. Make up a solution of the drug (1 g chlormethiazole in 500 ml 5% glucose solution). Load the patient with 50–100 ml of the drug solution until the seizure is aborted. Continue to infuse drug at a rate of 5–15 ml/hr after the seizures are aborted.
10. In cases where there seizure is resistant to all abortive therapy, consider induction of barbiturate coma

(thiopentone 50 to 100 mg bolus −3 to 5 mg/kg/hr infusion). The treatment should be decided by a neurologist, and performed in ICU. EEG monitoring is required, and the patient required intubation.

Maintenance therapy

11. As soon as the patient is given abortive therapy, maintenance therapy should also be started immediately.

    (i) Phenytoin. The drug is given as a slow (over 20–60 minutes) bolus injection. The dose is 15–20 mg/kg body weight. Monitor heart rate and blood pressure when this drug is given. If there is hypotension or bradycardia, reduce the rate of injection. Avoid extravasation.

    (ii) Fosphenytoin. Phenytoin solution will be phased out over the next few months. The dose and manner in which Fosphenytoin is given is the same as phenytoin. Hypotension and bradycardia is less common, but monitoring is still required.

    (iii) Sodium valproate. This drug is given as a slow bolus (over 15–30 minutes). The usual loading dose is 10–20 mg/kg body weight. This drug should be avoided in patients known to have hepatic dysfunction.

12. Once the patient is adequate stabilised and investigated, definitive management plan should be formulated. Long term anticonvusant therapy is usually needed. Refer to neurology service.

GASTROINTESTINAL

ACUTE DIARRHOEA
LIM SENG GEE

Definition

Acute diarrhoea < 3 weeks duration.

Clinical evaluation

Almost always due to infection, but other diagnoses should be considered. Evaluate hydration status.

1. Diarrhoea + vomitting (food poisoning) — within hours of contaminated meal/food, no fever, diarrhoea watery/unformed, short duration (24 hrs); caused by preformed toxin: *Staph. aureus, Bacillus cereus, Clostr. perfringens.*

2. Watery diarrhoea (may be large volume) — usually 1–2 days after contaminated food/water, no fever, large volume diarrhoea may occur — danger of dehydration; diarrhoea continues despite fasting; can last up to 1 week; caused by toxins: cholera, ETEC.

3. Diarrhoea + fever — usually 1–2 days after contaminated food/water, diarrhoea may be non-specific or have blood ± mucous; lasts from days to wks; caused by invasive organisms: Shigella, Salmonella, Amoeba, Yersenia, Campylobacter (pain++), EIAC.

4. Bloody diarrhoea — similar to above, but clear cut colitis will need to consider other possible DDx: acute inflammatory bowel disease, TB gut, ischaemic colitis (elderly).

5. Bulky/greasy stools (steatorrhoea) — acute presentation suggest giardia, but tropical sprue and Whipple's are rare causes.

6. Non-specific diarrhoea — loose stools without any of above features. Have to exclude all possible pathogens.

Special circumstances

1. Traveller's diarrhoea — during or shortly after travelling; may have any of the above patterns; usually due to ETEC, salmonella, giardia and amoeba.

2. Diarrheoa in homosexuals — have to differentiate

mucous and pus PR from true diarrhoea; mucous and pus due to rectal gonorrhoea, syphillis, lymphogranuloma venerum; diarrhoea due to amoeba, giardia, shigella.

3. Diarrhoea in HIV pts — helpful if CD4 counts are known (pts usually know their counts): CD4 > 200 — likely to have acute self limiting diarrhoea, have to consider all of the acute infections including cryptosporida and amoeba; CD < 200 — acute diarrhoea likely to become chronic, likelihood of pathogen if diarrhoea is severe ± wt loss, probable pathogens are cryptosporidia, microsporidia, CMV, giardia, amoeba.

4. Diarrhoea in hospitalised pts or pts recently on antibiotics with fever, ± blood, ± mucous: exclude pseudomembranous colitis; consider drugs — laxatives, antacids, colchicine, theophylline, digitalis, NSAIDs; consider excessive nasogastric or nasoenteric feeds; note that nosocomial outbreaks of ETEC, EIAC, *Clostr. difficile* may occur.

Diarrhoea associated with medical illnesses

1. Chemotherapy/transplant pts — consider pseudomembranous colitis, mucositis, GVHD (esp BMT) and drugs.

2. Rheumatic disease/SLE — if associated with sacroilietis or arthritis, consider inflammatory bowel disease with seronegative arthropathy. Also Reiter's if uveitis or urethritis. If SLE, consider vasculitis (usually with PR bleeding/bloody diarrhoea).

3. Post abdominal surgery — dumping syndrome post Billroth II, bacterial overgrowth if blind loop, bile salt malabsorption post-terminal ileal resection.

4. Endocrine diseases — autonomic neuropathy in diabetics, increased GI motility in thyrotoxicosis.

Investigations:
1. FBC, electrolytes, urea and creatinine, WWF.
2. Stools for culture; ova, cysts and parasites; occult blood; fat smear (if indicated); C difficile toxin.

3. Blood cultures if febrile.
4. Stool electrolytes and osmolality for chronic diarrhoea.

Management
1. If large volume watery diarrhoea, admit, fast and start IV fluids for rehydration.
2. Start ciprofloxacin 250mg bd for 1 week (including traveller's diarrhoea), except in those cases of special circumstances listed above.
3. Remember that most cases of acute diarrhoea settle within 1 week.
4. If diarrhoea has not settled within 1 week in hospital, and investigations are negative, colonoscopy should be considered.
5. Other investigations to be considered if indicated (usually if diarrhoea becomes chronic): OGD + jejenal biopsies, small bowel enema, 3-day fecal fat collection, stool electrolytes and osmolality.

GASTROINTESTINAL HAEMORRHAGE
LIM SENG GEE

Clinical presentation
Haematemesis, malaena and fresh PR bleeding.

Important points to remember
1. Ensure patient is clinically stable before pursuing further history and examination.
2. Most malaena and fresh PR bleeding are due to upper GI causes and hence OGD should be performed first.

Relevant clinical features

clinical features	*cause*
PHx peptic ulcer or ulcer surgery	peptic ulcer
epigastric pain assoc. with meals	peptic ulcer
NSAID usage	NSAID enteropathy
PHx liver disease, drinking, ascites	varices
Recurrent vomiting	Mallory weiss tear
significant weight loss	GI malignancy

Clinical evaluation
1. Check the vitals.
2. Look for signs of liver disease: jaundice, spider naevi, palmar erythema, gynaecomastia, liver flap, leukonychia, clubbing, ascites.
3. Abdominal mass.
4. PR to confirm malaena.
5. Assess severity of GI bleed — > 1L blood loss: tachycardia > 100, postural hypotension, BP < 100, cool and clammy extremities.

Diagnostic considerations in GI bleeding

Upper GI bleeding	Lower GI bleeding
bleeding from nose/pharynx	haemorrhoids
hemoptysis	anal fissure
esophageal tear (Mallory-Weiss)	inflammatory bowel disease
esophageal ulceration/tumour	neoplasm: Ca or polyps
haemorrhagic gastric erosions: NSAIDs, renal failure, stress	diverticular disease
peptic ulcer of stomach, duo	ischaemic enteritis/colitis
Dieulafoy's lesion (ruptured mucosal artery)	angiodysplasia
varices of esophagus, stomach	antibiotic related colitis
gastric neoplasm: Ca, lymphoma, leiomyoma, polyps	radiation colitis
haemobilia	meckel's diverticulum
vascular-enteric fistula (AA repair)	infective colitis: amoeba

Management

1. Two large bore IV cannula.
2. Resuscitate patient as a priority: IV normal saline, colloid (haemacel) in preference to normal saline, and fresh blood in preference to colloid or packed cells. In the presence of clinically significant GI bleeding, at least 3 units of blood should be given as blood loss > 1,000 mls.
3. Correct coagulopathy (FFP).
4. Give platelets if platelet count < 80,000 or patient has been on NSAIDs in the absence of an ulcer.
5. Consider IV somatostatin (250 μg/hour is useful in the first 48 hours of GI bleed, esp. for varices).
6. Give H_2-blockers (iv ranitidine 50 mg q8hrs) or proton-channel blockers (iv omeprazole 40 mg om).
7. Urgent OGD (injection, heater probe, super-glue, or band ligation), contact on-call endoscopist.

8. If OGD is normal, then urgent colonoscopy should be performed.
9. If colonoscopy is normal or no cause is found despite careful examination, then bleeding labelled RBC GI bleeding scan should be performed if bleeding is still active (need blood loss of 0.1 ml/min to have a positive result). This can only localise the lesion approximately. Coeliac axis or mesenteric angiogram can localise the lesion more precisely if there is active bleeding of 0.5–1 ml/min.
10. If bleeding is massive, consider intubation for airway protection.
11. Minnesota tube or Sengstaken-Blakemore tube can be inserted for variceal bleeing.
12. Refer to surgeon if bleeding continues for surgical option.

ACUTE LIVER FAILURE
LO SU KONG and LEE KANG HOE

Definition: Development of encephalopathy in a patient who has no pre-existing symptomatic liver disease. Many different time scales have been used.

King's College Hospital criteria:
1. Hyperacute: encephalopathy within 7 days of jaundice.
2. Acute: encephalopathy 8 to 28 days from onset of jaundice.
3. Subacute: encephalopathy 4–12 weeks from the onset of jaundice.

Clinical evaluation
1. Assess vitals — check airway. Grade the encephalopathy (Grade 0: Normal; Grade 1: Drowsy but oriented; Grade 2: Drowsy and disorientated; Grade 3: Un-cooperative, agitated, shouting, screaming, behavioral changes (aggressive); Grade 4: Coma). Note any eye signs or focal neurology.
2. Examine for stigmata of chronic liver disease.
3. Look for cause of liver failure (in particular drug history, blood transfusions, sexual history, travel, previous hepatitis).
4. Complications from liver failure: infection (spontaneous bacterial peritonitis, pneumonia, urinary tract infection); bleeding; renal failure; hypoglycemia; acidosis; cerebral oedema; ascites.

Mortality related to grade of encephalopathy: Grade 1–2: < 20%; Grade 3–4: > 80%.

Some causes of acute liver failure (ALF)
1. Viral hepatitis: Hep A — IgM antibody; Hep B — IgM core antibody (co-infection or superinfection with delta agent can present as ALF); Hep C — usually seen in patients

with chronic liver diseases. Unusual cause of ALF; Hep D — IgM antibody; Hep E — IgG/IgM antibody. High mortality in pregnant patients; Non A — E (or indeterminate) hepatitis; Other viruses (EBV etc).
2. Drug induced (some examples only): Anti-TB (Isoniazid + Rifampicin); Anti-epileptics (phenytoin, carbamazepine); Halothane; Cloxacillin; Paracetomol.
3. Acute fatty liver of pregnancy: third trimester, hypoglycaemia, raised uric acid, disseminated intravascular coagulopathy.
4. Others: lymphoma; Wilson's disease, alcholic, Budd-Chiari syndrome.

Investigations

1. Blood investigations: FBC, electrolytes, urea and creatinine, liver function test, DIC screen, FactorV level, lactate, ABG, ammonia, X-match, blood cultures, hepatitis markers (HAV, HBsAg, Anti-HBs, Anti-HBc, HBeAg, Anti-HBe, HBV DNA, HCV, Delta antigen), Wilson's disease (serum caeruloplasmin, urine copper), toxicology (include paracetamol level).
2. Imaging: CXR, Ultrasound of liver and Doppler of vessels (portal vein, hepatic vein and artery), CT abdomen, CT head if focal neurology or Grade 4 encephalopathy.
3. Culture sputum, urine, ascitic fluid (if SBP).

Management

1. General measures: minimal tactile stimulation; monitor airway control; try nursing 10° head-up; oxygen supplementation.
2. Nutrition: NG if possible (no documented advantage of branch-chained amino-acids), otherwise TPN. Protein 40G per day — may be increased once patient is no longer encephalopathic. Vitamin supplement (include vitamin K 10 mg for 3 days).
3. Correct electrolytes abnormalities, and watch for hypoglycemia.

4. Antifungals: Nystatin 500,000 units qid orally; iv amphotericn B for those meeting liver transplantation (TP) criteria, renal failure and grade 4 encephalopathy, high risk repeat TP, or those ventilated with broad spectrum antibiotics and still febrile.

5. Antibiotics: iv Unasyn (alternative iv cefuroxime) as first line for 5 days, unless specific culture results dictate otherwise.

6. Stress ulcer prophylaxis: sucralfate 2 g qid oral.

7. Maintain intravascular volume to reduce risk of renal failure.

8. Do not correct PT with FFP unless bleeding or for invasive procedure. PT allows monitoring of liver function.

9. Invasive lines as dictated by hemodynamic condition. Beware of coagulopathy (lines can be inserted with careful technique despite high PT), and risk of infection.

10. Intubate and ventilate patients that cannot protect their airway, have significant GI bleeding, or in Grade 3 or 4 encephalopathy.

11. Head chart monitoring: monitor for raised intracranial pressure — intracranial pressure monitoring, and jugular bulb oximetry. Treat with 100 to 200 ml of 20% mannitol if raised ICP (Keep serum osmolality < 310 mmol/L). Consider hemofiltration if renal failure, and barbiturate coma. EEG monitoring.

12. Specific treatment for underlying disease if possible: HBV DNA positive — lamivudine (experimental — especially if listed for liver transplantation).

13. Liver transplantation should be considered early before patient is too ill or infected (refer early to liver transplant centre at NUH).

Criteria for listing for liver transplantation (not paracetamol)

1. PT > 100 seconds — irrespective of anything else.

2. Any three of the following: (i) age < 10 or > 40; (ii) aetiolgy (Non A non B, halothane, drugs); (iii) jaundice > 7 days

before encephalopathy; (iv) PT > 50 secs; (v) Bilirubin > 300 mmol/l.

Paracetamol overdose: (i) Arterial pH < 7.3 or (ii) the presence of all the following: prothrombin time > 100 secs, Grade 3/4 encephalopathy, creatinine > 300 mmol/l.

LIVER FAILURE IN CIRRHOTICS
LO SU KONG

Causes
1. Infection (consider spontaneous bacterial peritonitis).
2. Gastro-intestinal bleeds.
3. Excessive protein intake.
4. Dehydration (over-diuresis)/urea/electrolyte imbalance.
5. Drugs — sedatives.
6. Constipation.

Clinical evaluation
See acute liver failure.

Investigations
1. FBC, PT/PTT, electrolytes, urea and creatinine, LFT, glucose level, ammonia, X-match.
2. Septic workup: blood cultures and other appropriate cultures.
3. CXR.
4. Ascites tap (spontaneous bacterial peritonitis: neutrophils > 250/mm^3 or total WBC > 500/mm^3) — culture fluid in blood culture bottles.
5. Oesophago-gastro-duodenoscopy if indicated.

Management
1. Vital signs monitoring.
2. Urine output.
3. Blood sugar monitoring.
4. Daily weights.
5. Encephalopathy: lactulose — aim for 2 soft stools per day (avoid diarrhoea); low protein diet — 40 g to 60 g protein daily; enema; consider metronidazole; consider neomycin.
6. Spontaneous bacterial peritonitis — antibiotic choices: Unasyn 1.5 G tid iv or Ciprofloxacin 200 mg bid iv.
7. As for acute liver failure.
8. Consider liver transplantation if appropriate.

ACUTE HEPATOBILIARY SEPSIS
YEOH KHAY GUAN

Acute infections of the hepatobiliary system include: cholangitis, cholecystitis, empyema of the gallbladder, and liver abscess.

Pathophysiology

Cholangitis, cholecystitis and empyema of the gallbladder most often occur secondary to gallstones. Cholangitis occurs due to partial or complete obstruction to bile flow, and bacteria are present in bile-culture in 75% of cases. Acute cholecystitis is due to acute inflammation of the gallbladder following obstruction of the cystic duct by a stone. Empyema of the gallbladder results from progression of acute cholecystitis due to superinfection by a pyogenic organism, and carries a high risk of septicemia and perforation.

Liver abscess can be caused by pyogenic organisms or amoebiasis. Most cases of liver abscess in Singapore are pyogenic abscesses. The commonest aetiological organism is *Klebsiella pneumonia*. Other causative organisms include: other gram negative bacteria, staphylococci and anaerobes. Meliodosis is also a cause in endemic countries like Thailand. Suspect amoebic liver abscess if there has recent travel to developing countries or if the patient is an immigrant from such countries.

Clinical evaluation

1. Cholecystitis: Fever, chills, rigors, biliary colic, vomiting, right hypochondrial tenderness, progressing to severe RHC tenderness and septicemia in empyema.
2. Cholangitis: biliary colic, jaundice, fever (Charcot's triad). Suppurative acute cholangitis is a medical emergency because pus production in an obstructed biliary system rapidly progresses to septicemia and shock.
3. Liver abscess: Fever, chills and rigors, right hypochondrial pain and tenderness. Presentation in the elderly may be atypical and a high index of suspicion is required.

Investigations
1. FBC, urea, electrolytes and creatinine, liver function tests.
2. Blood cultures x 3 before starting antibiotics.
3. Urgent ultrasound abdomen (within 24 hours).

The presence of obstructive jaundice in combination with sepsis indicates cholangitis, and urgent biliary drainage by ERCP may be required.

Management
1. Nil-by-mouth, IV antibiotics, i.v. hydration, correct electrolytes (patient frequently vomiting), analgesia (pethidine preferable, avoid morphine as this causes spasm of the sphincter of Oddi), hourly parameters.
2. Antibiotic choice for biliary sepsis: If the patient is young and has normal renal function: IV ampicillin 500 mg to 1 g 6 hourly and IV gentamicin 3–4.5 mg/kg/day in 3 divided doses and IV metronidazole 500 mg 8 hourly. If the patient is elderly or aminoglycosides contraindicated: IV ampicillin/sulbactam (Unasyn) 1.5 g 6 hourly or IV ceftriaxone 2 g daily, and IV metronidazole 500 mg 8 hourly. If penicillin-sensitive, substitute with IV ciprofloxacin 200 mg 12 hourly. For liver abscesses, a similar combination is appropriate, and metronidazole is useful as it covers both amoebiasis as well as anaerobes.

3. Particular considerations:
   (i) Cholangitis: Biliary drainage by ERCP or PTC usually necessary if obstruction persists.
   (ii) Cholecystitis: Initial treatment with IV antibiotics, deferring cholecystectomy till when inflammation has subsided, unless patient fails to improve with antibiotics.
   (iii) If empyema of the gallbladder is suspected, emergency surgical intervention with appropriate antibiotic coverage is required.

ACUTE PANCREATITIS
LIM SENG GEE

Pathophysiology

Acute inflammatory process involving the pancreas and other retroperitoneal tissues. Fat necrosis, oedema, and infiltration of the pancreas with inflammatory cells. Systemic upset occurs if severe with manifestations of SIRS.

Presents with

1. Acute abdominal pain — epigastric, sharp, radiating to back. Can have rigid abdomen. Discolouration around the umbilicus (Cullen's sign).
2. Vomiting
3. May have shock if severe.
   Look for history of cholelithiasis, alcohol, steroids, diuretics, abdominal surgery, trauma, ERCP.

Diagnosis

1. Clinical
2. Blood tests: serum amylase (> 1000 IU/ml) (75%), serum lipase (70%), both (80–85%) — remains elevated for 3–5 days.
3. Urine amylase remains elevated for 7–10days.
4. Radiology:
   (i) AXR — ileus, exclude perforated viscus, absent psoas shadow owing to retroperitoneal fluid,
   (ii) CT scan abdo — oedematous pancreas, necrotic/ haemorrhagic areas in pancreas, peripancreatic fluid or air. (Note that a normal CT abdo does not exclude pancreatitis, but makes the likelihood of severe pancreatitis unlikely.)

Ranson's criteria for evaluating severity (≥ 3 considered severe)

(i) On admission: age > 55 years, WBC > 16,000/mm^3, hyperglycemia, LDH > 350 IU/L, AST > 250 IU/L.

(ii) During initial 48 hours: Hct decrease > 10%, increase in urea, fall in calcium, hypoxemia, increased base deficit, fluid sequestration of > 6 litres.

Investigations
1. Blood investigations: ABG, FBC, PT/PTT, electrolytes, urea and creatinine, LFT, Ca^{2+}, Mg, amylase, lipids, X-match.
2. Imaging: AXR and CT abdomen (Ultra-sound is an option if patient is too ill to transport).

Management
1. IV cannulas x 2.
2. Resuscitation — general supportive measures. Fluid resuscitation required as large volumes lost within the abdomen. May require central pressure monitoring. Electrolyte imbalances should be corrected (hypocalcemia and hypomagnesemia). Oxygen supplementation including mechanical ventilation as required, especially if ARDS develops. Consider ICU admission.
3. Watch urine output (> 0.5 ml/kg/hr) — may require urinary catheterisation.
4. Analgesia — pethidine 50 to 100 mg IM.
5. NG tube and nil by mouth.
6. Attempts to reduce pancreatic secretion — iv somatostatin 250 g stat and 250 g/hr.
7. Peritoneal lavage in certain severe pancreatitis, especially if hemorrhagic.
8. Acute ERCP if obstruction present from biliary stone — improves outcome.
9. Prophylactic antibiotics — controversial. Cover for gram-negative enteric organisms.
10. Look out for complications: infection/abscess, pseudocyst formation (persistently elevated amylase), diabetes, multi-organ failure — renal failure, DIVC, ARDS. Percutaneous drainage of infected pancreatic pseudocysts can be attempted.
11. If fasting becomes prolonged, consider TPN.

INFECTIOUS DISEASES

SEPSIS (SIRS) AND SHOCK
LEE KANG HOE

The body responds to infection in a standard systemic fashion. This reaction may also be induced by non-infectious causes and has therefore been labelled as SIRS (systemic inflammatory response syndrome). This includes 2 or more of the following:

1) Temperature $> 38°C$ or $< 36°C$,
2) Heart rate > 90 bpm,
3) Respiratory rate > 20 breaths/min or $PaCO_2 < 32$ mmHg,
4) White cell count $> 12.0 \times 10^9/L$ or $< 4.0 \times 10^9/L$ or the presence of more than 10% immature neutrophils.

Therefore, other causes of SIRS besides sepsis include trauma, pancreatitis, burns, IL-2 therapy.

Sepsis is SIRS with a documented infection. Severe sepsis is now defined as the presence of sepsis with hypotension (systolic BP < 90 mmHg or reduction > 40 mmHg from baseline) or systemic manifestations of hypoperfusion (mental obtundation, chest pain, hypoxemia, oliguria, metabolic acidosis, lactic acidosis). Septic shock is sepsis-induced hypotension despite fluid resuscitation plus hypotension abnormalities.

Mortality rates increase in a stepwise fashion: SIRS (7%), sepsis (16%), severe sepsis (20%), and septic shock (46%).

Hypotension develops from peripheral vasodilatation and possibility myocardial depression, secondary to increased production of nitric oxide.

The management of sepsis requires prompt identification of the responsible organism and the site of sepsis, while providing good supportive therapy.

Management

1. A history, physical examination, laboratory investigations, ECG, appropriate cultures, and radiological imaging are required. Document evidence of hypoperfusion.

2. Once cultures are taken, empiric choices of antibiotics (or specific treatment) should be administered.

3. Drainage of pus is required if possible (surgical or percutaneous).

4. Supportive care — assess vital signs or a regular basis, at least 2 large bore iv cannulae, provide supplemental oxygen, check urine output and conscious level, give adequate iv fluids.

5. IV fluids — patients are usually vasodilated and preload falls. They usually require large volume fluid resuscitation — central pressure monitoring is advised. Fluids should be isotonic. Give up to 2 litres of crystalloid (Normal saline or Lactated Ringer's) initially — check for fluid overload, and BP/HR response. Consider colloids (PPF or Hetastarch 7%) if still hypovoloemic. If adequately loaded (CVP 12 to 15 or PAWP 12 to 18 mmHg), then consider the commencement of inotropes (Dopamine 5 ug/kg/min). Titrate according to BP response.

6. Continual reassessment is required. Check for resolution of metabolic acidosis, urine output, mental status and blood pressure. If patient continues to deteriorate, consider ICU admission and elective intubation with invasive hemodynamic monitoring.

7. Choice of inotropes — Dopamine should the first choice. Once, a dose of 20 ug/kg/min is reached and the patient is still hypotensive, consider commencement of noradrenaline (start at 0.05 ug/kg/min) or adrenaline (start at 0.05 ug/kg/min). A cardiac output should be performed to ensure an adequate cardiac index (> 2.0 L/min/m^2). Dopamine should either be discontinued or reduced to low dose ranges for putative renal vasodilatation (2 to 5 ug/kg/min). If CI is inadequate, dobutamine can be added to noradrenaline. If adrenaline is already employed, there is no additional benefit for adding dobutamine.

8. Consider adrenal insufficiency if patient becomes totally unresponsive to inotropes.

9. Ensure acid-base is corrected and ionised calcium levels are adequate.
10. If patient becomes asystolic on high-dose inotropes, it is futile to commence CPR.
11. Note that the optimal management of sepsis is to prevent the development of shock. Thus, prompt and adequate fluid resuscitation is important.

ANTIBIOTICS FOR COMMON INFECTIONS
TI TEOW YEE and TAN CHORH CHUAN

A. Urinary tract infections (UTI)

Cystitis

Clinical evaluation
Dysuria, frequency, ± gross haematuria, low grade fever. Presence of these symptoms without flank pain does not exclude pyelonephritis.

Investigations
FBC, urine microscopy for pyuria, urine culture and sensitivity.

Management
1. Community-acquired, non-pregnant female:
   (i) If culture shows susceptible organism, oral Amoxycillin 500 mg tds × 3 days, otherwise/or,
   (ii) Trimethoprim 100 mg tds × 3 days (or trimethoprim-sulphamethoxazole 2 tab bd × 3 days), or, Nitrofurantoin 50 mg qds × 5 days.
2. Hospital-acquired, non-pregnant female: Ciprofloxacin 250–500 mg bd × 1 week, or Pefloxacin 400 mg bd × 1 week.
3. Male patients with cystitis: Same antibiotics as above but for a minimum of 10–14 days.

Acute pyelonephritis

Clinical evaluation
High fever ± chills and rigors, loin pain or backache, dysuria, frequency and urgency.

Investigations
FBC, urine microscopy for pyuria, urine and blood culture (before starting antibiotics).

Management
1. Community-acquired:
   (i) If patient is young and has no renal impairment: IV Ampicillin 2 g 6 hourly and IV gentamicin 3–4.5 mg/kg/day in 2 or 3 divided doses.
   (ii) If patient allergic to beta lactams, gentamicin alone is usually adequate.
   (iii) If patient is old or aminoglycosides are contra-indicated, give: IV cefuroxime 750 mg 8 hourly, or IV ciprofloxacin 100–200 mg 12 hourly, or IV Ampicillin/Sulbactam (Unasyn) 1.5 g 8 hourly, or Amoxycillin/Clavulanate (Augmentin) 1.2 g 8 hourly.

2. Hospital-acquired or complicated UTI (renal stones, urine catheter, obstruction):
   (i) IV ceftazidime 1 g 8 hourly, or IV ciprofloxacin 100–200 mg 12 hourly
   (ii) If patient critically ill, and no contraindication to aminoglycosides, add IV amikacin 7.5 mg/kg 12 hourly (if renal function normal).
   (iii) Remove urine catheter if possible and relieve ureteral obstruction.

Catheter associated UTI
Significant bacterial growth is usual in the urine of patients with indwelling urine catheters for more than a few days.

Do not treat these patients unless there are symptoms and signs to suggest systemic infection. Prolonged or repeated courses of antibiotics to treat urine culture reports are usually not effective in sterilising urine as long as the catheter is in situ, and would select out multiresistant organisms and fungi.

Candiduria

In patients who have received broad-spectrum antibiotics or with indwelling urine catheters, it is not uncommon to isolate candida from the urine.

This is NOT an indication to initiate anti-fungal therapy.

Consultation should be sought to decide on the need for antifungal treatment.

B. Biliary tract infections

Biliary tract infections include cholecystitis, cholangitis and empyema of the gallbladder.

Clinical evaluation
1. Usual presentation: high fever, right hypochondrial pain or biliary colic, obstructive jaundice.
2. Abdominal symptoms and signs may be minimal especially in the elderly.

Investigations
1. FBC, electrolytes, urea and creatinine, liver function tests
2. Septic workup: blood culture × 3 before starting antibiotics.
3. Urgent ultrasound abdomen.

Management
1. Nil-by-mouth, IV hydration, hourly parameters.
2. If the patient is young and has normal renal function: IV Ampicillin 1 g 6 hourly and IV Gentamicin 3–4.5 mg/kg/day in 2 or 3 divided doses and IV Metronidazole 500 mg 8–12 hourly.
3. If patient elderly or aminoglycosides contraindicated: IV Ampicillin/Sulbactam (Unasyn) 1.5 g 6 hourly, or IV Ceftriaxone 1 g daily and IV Metronidazole 500 mg 8–12 hourly.
4. Decompression by PTC or ERCP if obstruction present.

C. Diabetic foot infections

Clinical evaluation

Diabetic foot infections should ALWAYS be taken seriously and treated aggressively. They may be classified as:

1. Non limb-threatening infections: No systemic signs of sepsis, superficial lesions, minimal cellulitis
2. Limb-threatening infections: Extensive cellulitis, lymphangitis, deep ulcers, ± fever, necrotising fasciitis (if extension deep and proximal).

Investigations

1. FBC, electrolytes, urea and creatinine, HbA1c.
2. Septic workup: blood culture × 3 for moderate to severe infections, swab of ulcer (pus) for Gram stain and culture.
3. X-ray of limb — look for underlying osteomyelitis or gas in subcutaneous tissue.

Management

1. Non limb-threatening infections (previously untreated) — usually streptococci and staphylococci. Oral Amoxycillin 500 mg 8 hourly and Cloxacillin 500 mg 6 hourly, or oral Cephalexin 500 mg 6 hourly.
2. Limb-threatening infections — infection usually polymicrobial with aerobes and anaerobes. IV Cloxacillin 1 g 6 hourly and IV Ceftriaxone 0.5–1 g 12 hourly and IV Metronidazole 500 mg 12 hourly.
3. Modify antibiotic treatment when culture results available.
4. Referral to Orthopaedic service for surgical debridement.
5. Maintain blood sugar < 10 mmol/l pre-meals with soluble insulin tds.

D. Cellulitis

Community-acquired cellulitis is usually due to Streptococcus pyogenes or Staphylococcus aureus.

1. If early or mild: Oral Cloxacillin 500 mg 6 hourly or Erythromycin 250–500 mg qds.
2. If more severe: IV Cloxacillin 1 g 6 hourly and IV Crystalline Penicillin 1 MU 6 hourly.

E. Malaria

Plasmodium vivax
Oral Chloroquine 600 mg base then 300 mg base 6 hours later, then 300 mg base om for 2 days + Primaquine 15 mg base om for 14 days. If patient is pregnant or G6PD-deficient, refer to ID specialist as the management is difficult. Primaquine should not be given during pregnancy. Primaquine may cause hemolysis in patients with G6PD-deficiency.

Plasmodium falciparum
Malaria caused by P. falciparum in most parts of the world is now resistant to chloroquine. Monitor response to treatment with daily percentage count of parasite load. Check G6PD status.

1. Uncomplicated P Falciparum malaria:
   (i) Oral Quinine sulphate 600 mg salt tds × 3–7 days and Tetracycline 250 mg qds × 7 days., or
   (ii) Oral Mefloquine 20 mg/kg mefloquine base as a single dose (to maximum 1.5 g) — (note: may cause central nervous system adverse effects, e.g. neuropsychiatric disturbances, circulatory abnormalities, e.g. tachycardia and conduction disorders).

2. Patient cannot take orally or severely ill (impaired consciousness, severe anaemia, renal failure, jaundice, pulmonary oedema, DIC, shock, hypoglycaemia, repeated seizures, parasitaemia > 5%):
   (i) Manage in ICU as mortality may be up to 30%, may require mechanical ventilation,
   (ii) IV Quinine dihydrochloride 20 mg salt/kg loading dose (to maximum 1.4 g) in 5% dextrose over 4 hours, THEN after 8–12 hours, IV 10 mg salt/kg

(to maximum 750 mg)over 4 hours every 8–12 hours, until patient can take orally.

(iii) Can consider red-cell exchange transfusion if parasite load is high (> 5%) and patient has cerebral malaria.

MELIOIDOSIS

Melioidosis is caused by Burkholderia pseudomallei.

Clinical evaluation

1. Manifestations range from subclinical to septicaemic infection.
2. In the septicaemic form, abscesses can develop in the skin, lungs, liver, spleen, prostate, and lymph nodes. The mortality rate associated with severe septicaemic infection is 85–95%.
3. The infection is characterised by a high relapse rate.

Investigations

1. FBC,electrolytes, urea and creatinine, liver function tests.
2. Septic workup: blood culture × 3 before starting antibiotics, sputum, urine, and wound cultures,.
3. Imaging: CXR, abdominal ultrasound or CT, bone imaging as indicated.

Management

The organism is generally susceptible to chloramphenicol, tetracycline, ceftazidime, piperacillin, imipenem, and amoxicillin/clavulanate.

(i) Mild to moderately severe infection, patient clinically stable: IV Ceftazidime 100 mg/kg/day in 2–3 divided doses (maximum 6 g/day),

(ii) Severe infection and patient is critically ill: IV Ceftazidime as above and IV Chloramphenicol 500 mg 6–8 hourly; If the infection cannot be controlled, a third antibiotic may be indicated.

(iii) Abscesses should be drained if they are accessible and large enough.

PNEUMONIA

LEE KANG HOE and LIM TOW KEANG

Diagnosis: cough with sputum and a fever (>38°C), and a new infiltrate on the chest radiograph (exclude heart failure, chronic lung disease, and tumour).

Community-acquired if acquired within 48 hours of admission and admitted from home. Nosocomial, if recent hospitalisation (≤ 30 days) or from nursing home.

Community-acquired pneumonia

Divide into non-immunocompromised and immunocompromised.

Evaluate patients for severity category (ATS Guidelines 1993):
1. Outpatient — ≤ 60 years with no comorbid disease.
2. Outpatient — > 60 years with comorbid disease.
3. In-hospital.
4. Severe pneumonia — usually ICU.

Criteria for hospital admission: RR ≥ 30 bpm, SBP < 90 mm Hg, pulse ≥ 125/min, temperature < 35°C or 40°C, evidence of extrapulmonary sites of disease, confusion, comorbid disease (chronic lung disease, DM, renal failure, heart failure, liver cirrhosis, alcoholic, malnourished, postsplenectomy), or laboratory abnormalities (see below), inability to take oral medications, poor social support.

Laboratory evidence of increased morbidity and mortality:
1. WBC < 4×10^9/L or > 30×10^9/L or an absolute neutrophil count < 1×10^9/L,
2. PaO_2 < 60 mm Hg or $PaCO_2$ > 50 mm Hg on room air, or pulse oximetry < 90%,
3. Urea > 7 mmol/L,
4. Hb < 9 g/dl,
5. Arterial pH < 7.35,

6. CXR — pleural effusion, more than 1 lobe involvement, presence of cavity, and rapid radiographic spreading.

Criteria for ICU admission (severe pneumonia): PaO_2/FiO_2 ratio < 250 (hypoxemia), respiratory fatigue/distress, shock, drowsiness/airway protection, oliguria.

Aetiology
Responsible pathogen not identified in 50%. Clinical and radiographic features are not diagnostic for specific pathogens. There may also be more than one pathogen.

Commonest: Strep pneumoniae, mycoplasma, H influenzae, viruses, Moraxella. Be aware of staph aureus, gram-negative bacilli (especially meliodosis) — especially in diabetics, TB, legionella.

For immunocompromised host, consider other organisms in the differential diagnosis: PCP, fungal, TB and viral.

Investigations
1. Laboratory investigations: FBC, electrolytes, urea and creatinine, liver function tests, ABG, Mycoplasma and Legionella serologies.
2. Radiology: CXR (PA ± lateral), occasionally CT thorax can be helpful.
3. Cultures: sputum (gram stain, look for AFB and perform TB cultures), blood, BAL (± TBB) if immunocompromised host.

Management
1. Supplemental oxygen (high flow). Respiratory failure will require ventilatory support.
2. If in shock, resuscitate.
3. Antibiotics (based on the categorization of patients clinical severity):
   Category 1: macrolide (erythromycin 500 mg qid po or EES 800 mg bid po; consider other macrolides — azithromycin or clarithromycin).

Category 2: second-generation cephalosporin (cefuroxime 500 mg bid po) or beta-lactam/beta-lactamase inhibitor (Unasyn ii bid po or Augmentin 375 mg tid po) plus/minus erythromycin).

Category 3: second or third generation cephalosporin (cefuroxime 750 mg tid iv or ceftriaxone 1G or 2G om iv) or beta-lactam/beta-lactamase inhibitor, plus or minus a macrolide.

Category 4: macrolide (erythromycin 500 mg qid iv) plus a third-generation cephalosporin with anti-pseudomonal activity (ceftazidime 2G bid iv) or a carbapenem, plus/minus staph aureus coverage (cloxacillin or vancomycin).

Immunocompromised: cover widely. Check HIV status is high-risk. Identify aetiologic agent urgently.

4. Consider anti-TB if chest radiograph is consistent and/or AFB positive.

Nosocomial pneumonia

Consider coverage of staph aureus (and MRSA) and gram-negative bacilli (beware of multi-resistance). May also require anaerobic coverage if obvious aspiration (beta-lactam/beta-lactamase inhibitor, or clindamycin). Preventive measures important (limit length of mechanical ventilation, don't feed if gag is absent, nurse head 30° to horizontal, be sparing in use of H_2-antagonists).

TUBERCULOSIS
LIM TOW KEANG

Introduction
The incidence of TB increases with age showing a sharp rise in the late teens to a peak in the elderly. Spread is via the respiratory tract and pulmonary TB (PTB) accounts for over 90% of new cases. To prevent the emergence of drug resistance, it is important to ensure compliance with treatment, which is best achieved by directly observed therapy (DOT).

Clinical evaluation and diagnosis
TB is diagnosed by:
1. Clinical presentation (intermittent fever, cough, weight loss),
2. Co-morbid conditions which may predispose to TB such as diabetes mellitus and silicosis including prior medication such as corticosteroids,
3. CXR — typical apical cavitation,
4. Microscopic examination of relevant specimens (AFB positive), and
5. Mycobacterial culture.

The tuberculin skin test is not a useful predictor of disease in Singapore because of previous BCG vaccination.

Further investigations:
1. Pleural biopsy in patients with exudative, lymphocyte rich pleural effusions.
2. Fiberoptic bronchoscopy to obtain lower respiratory secretions and lung tissue in patients with lung infiltrates.
3. Percutaneous image guided needle biopsy in patients with lung nodules.
4. Biopsy of enlarged regional lymph nodes.

5. More invasive studies such as open/thoraco-scopic mediastinal lymph node or lung biopsies may be indicated in selected patients with progressive disease.

In Singapore, routine cultures for *M. tuberculosis* are performed using a technique (Bactec) which return positive results within 2–3 weeks. Amplification of mycobacterial nucleic acid (either DNA or mRNA) using various molecular biology techniques may identify mycobacterial genes rapidly with reasonable accuracy. They should not, at the present time, be used in the routine diagnosis of TB.

TB is recognised as a defining illness in the AIDS syndrome. The majority of patients with TB in Singapore do not have AIDS. Testing for anti-HIV antibodies should be considered in all new patients with TB who present with atypical features such as wide dissemination, extensive lymph node and lower lung field disease.

Management
1. Isolation (ideally) for AFB positive patients.
2. Drug therapy.
3. Notifiable disease for contact tracing.

Drug therapy
In Singapore, 95% of all *M. tuberculosis* strains remained sensitive to streptomycin, isoniazid and rifampicin. Resistance to any single drug is < 5% and to multiple drugs < 1%. The basic principles of anti-TB treatment are (i) a combination of drugs — to prevent the emergence of resistance, and (ii) prolonged treatment — to eliminate slowly growing bacilli sequestrated in macrophages to prevent relapse.

Standard regimen: 2 month initial phase of isoniazid, rifampicin and pyrazinamide given daily followed by a continuation phase of 4 months of daily isoniazid and rifampicin.

Suspected drug resistance (e.g. non-residents and HIV +ve patients): 4 drugs (addition of ethambutol or streptomycin) should be started until the return of sensitivity results.

Non-infectious 2 weeks after starting treatment.

The cure rate with this regimen, in drug susceptible disease is 100% with relapse rates below 5%.

Side-effects: gastro-intestinal side effects are common; minor skin hypersensitivity reactions may be treated with anti-histamines; hepatitis is a rare but potentially fatal side effect of either isoniazid, rifampicin or pyrazinamide; patients on ethambutol — optic nerve screening for optic nerve disease and potential loss of colour vision.

Patients should be advised to stop all medication if they experience severe anorexia, nausea or jaundice. Serial LFT should be monitored in patients known to have liver dysfunction.

Except for streptomycin, (ototoxicity) which should never be used in pregnancy, no foetal toxicity is associated with the other first line anti-TB drugs and no dosage modification is needed in nursing mothers. The induction of liver enzymes by rifampicin may render oral contraceptive agents non-effective, and also lower cyclosporin or tacrolimus levels in transplant patients.

Drugs

1. Isoniazid   ≤ 40 kg   200 mg
                      > 40 kg   300 mg
   + Pyridoxine 10 mg/day in the elderly and malnourished.

2. Rifampicin   ≤ 50 kg   450 mg
                      > 50 kg   600 mg

3. Pyrazinamide   ≤ 50 kg   1.5 G
                      > 50 kg   2 G

4. Streptomycin   ≤ 50 kg   0.75 G
                      > 50 kg   1.5 G
   Avoid in renal failure.

5. Ethambutol   15 mg/kg
   Modify in renal failure.

ENDOCRINOLOGY

1. Diabetic ketoacidosis (DKA) and
   hyperosmolar hyperglycaemia
   non-ketoacidosis (HHNK)   *Thai AC*

2. Thyrotoxic crises (Thyroid storm)   *Cheah JS*

3. Myxoedema coma   *Cheah JS*

4. Adrenal insufficiency   *Lee KO*

5. Hypercalcaemia   *Chionh SB*

DIABETIC KETOACIDOSIS (DKA) AND HYPEROSMOLAR HYPERGLYCAEMIA NON-KETOACIDOSIS (HHNK)

THAI AH CHUAN

Definition

DKA and HHNK are diabetic emergencies characterised by:

1. Severe hyperglycaemia (blood glucose > 20 mmol/L but may be lower in some patients with DKA),
2. High serum osmolarity,
3. Additional diagnostic criteria for DKA include: pH < 7.35, low HCO_{3-}, high anion gap, urine ketones.

Clinical evaluation

1. Vital signs: BP, HR, conscious level (only 10% truly comatose), state of hydration.
2. Respiration: Kussmaul breathing from acidemia, may be depressed in severe acidosis.
3. Pyrexia: < 10% despite high incidence of infection. Hypo-thermia: usually mild with warm periphery.
4. Look for cause:
   (i) New-onset diabetics
   (ii) Known diabetics (80% identifiable factors): infection (UTI, pneumonia), AMI, stroke, pancreatitis, drugs, alcohol, trauma, treatment error, endocrine disorder.

Investigations

1. Bedside finger-prick blood glucose with portable glucose meter, and venous sample for laboratory estimation of plasma glucose.
2. FBC, electrolytes, urea and creatinine, ABG, CK and CKMB (as indicated).
3. Urine ketones, (plus plasma ketones if available).
4. ECG.
5. Septic workup: blood cultures, urine cultures, sputum cultures.
6. CXR.

Management

1. Fluid resuscitation: Normal saline initially (500–1000 mL NS per hour × 4 h); later if corrected serum $Na^+ >$ 150 mmol/L (250–500 mL 1/2 strength NS per hour × 4 hr), consider using 0.45% NaCl solution PROVIDED there is no hypotension. Monitor strict hourly intake-output, BP, pulse rate or CVP. Once blood glucose < 12 mmol/L, commence 5% glucose or dextrose/saline 500 mL 6–8 hourly. Saline infusion should continue for hydration as appropriate.

2. Insulin: IV soluble insulin 5–10 U bolus stat, then IV insulin by infusion pump: start at 6 U/hr (0.1 U/kg/hr); monitor blood glucose hourly and adjust rate 1–2 hourly to reduce blood glucose by 3–6 mmol/hour, till blood glucose is 12–14 mmol/l. Decrease insulin infusion rate, e.g. to 2–4 U/hr when blood glucose < 12 mmol/L aiming to keep blood glucose between 6–12 mmol/l. Monitor blood glucose 2–4 hourly. Subcutaneous insulin should only be given when patient takes oral diet well.

3. Correct electrolyte and acid-base balance: start K^+ replacement (40 mmol of 7.45% KCl solution) over an hour if serum K^+ < 3 mmol/L, 30 mmol over an hour if serum K^+ < 4 mmol/L, 20 mmol over an hour if serum K^+ < 5 mmol/L) as soon as possible based on electrolyte result; consider 4.2% or 8.4% sodium bicarbonate only if pH < 7.1, aiming to correct pH to 7.2.

4. Identify and reverse precipitating factors: appropriate antibiotics, or treat AMI, stroke, etc.

5. Intensive and continual monitoring: blood glucose with meter according to above schedule; send venous blood sample whenever meter reads 'HHH' and for every third meter reading for laboratory validation; serum Na^+, K^+, urea, creatinine, pH and blood gas every 1–4 hrs as appropriate.

6. Re-establish normal metabolism (recovery period)
    (i) Do not stop insulin. Stopping insulin as soon as blood glucose is at target value is a wrong practice! Blood glucose and ketone levels can rise rapidly

within 1–2 hrs of insulin withdrawal, with relapse of DKA and HHNK.

(ii)   Let patient eat as soon as he or she can.

(iii) If patient can tolerate oral diet, stop IV insulin infusion, and commence SC insulin e.g. regimen of soluble insulin before each meals and isophane (NPH) at bedtime. (NB: stop insulin infusion only 1–2 hrs after the first administration of SC short-acting insulin to allow for insulin level to peak.)

THYROTOXIC CRISES (THYROID STORM)
CHEAH JIN SENG

Definition
Thyrotoxic crisis or storm is a syndrome characterised by the triad of : fulminating increase in the symptoms and signs of thyrotoxicosis; hyperpyrexia; central nervous system manifestations (restlessness, delirium, coma).

Causes
1. Surgical: thyrotoxic patient undergoing thyroid surgery who is inadequately prepared for surgery, or surgery in patients with undiagnosed thyrotoxicosis.
2. Medical: in partially treated or untreated thyrotoxic patients, usually precipitated by complicating illness (usually sepsis) or a surgical emergency.

Clinical evaluation
1. High fever (often > 41°C).
2. Restlessness, confusion, clouding of consciousness, delirium, coma.
3. Vomiting, diarrhoea, signs of dehydration, hypotension.
4. Symptoms/signs of thyrotoxicosis: weight loss, sweatiness, tachycardia, goitre, exophthalmos.
5. Evaluate for irregular or partial treatment of thyrotoxicosis.
6. Symptoms/signs of precipitating cause (sepsis, trauma, surgical emergency, recent surgery).

Investigations
1. FBC, electrolytes, urea and creatinine, free thyroxine and TSH levels.
2. Septic workup: blood, sputum, and urine culture.
3. ECG.
4. CXR and other imaging as indicated.
5. Tests for suspected precipitating cause(s).

Management

1. Propylthiouracil loading dose 600–800 mg p.o., followed by p.o.100 mg every 2 hours; if patient unable to swallow, give through nasogastric tube. If vomiting present, give drug rectally as enema (same dose dissolved in Fleet's enema and administered via rectal tube with Nelaton balloon; retain for 2 hours).

2. IV Dexamethasone 2–4 mg 6–8 hourly.

3. IV sodium iodide 1 g in 500 ml of Normal Saline infused over 6 12 hours. Administer only AFTER PTU has been given for 1 hour, otherwise this may exacerbate the thyrotoxic state.

4. Propranolol p.o. 40–80 mg 6 hourly. In severe cases, propranolol may be given IV, e.g. 1–2mg over 5 mins (with ECG monitoring). If cardiac failure is present, digitalise before administering propranolol.

5. Correct dehydration if present, with IV Normal saline.

6. Treat precipitating cause, e.g. IV antibiotics for infection.

7. If patient is restless, sedate e.g. with chlorpromazine 25–50 mg IM or p.o.

8. Treat pyrexia with paracetamol and tepid sponging.

MYXOEDEMA COMA
CHEAH JIN SENG

Definition
Myxoedema coma is a severe form of hypothyroidism characterised by hypothermia, hyporeflexia, bradycardia, stupor
or coma, hypoventilation, hypoglycemia and fits. Not all
features need to be present for diagnosis. It is commoner
in the elderly in cold countries.

Causes
1. Hypothyroidism commonly due to surgery or radioiodine
   treatment for hyperthyroidism; autoimmune cause occasionally.
2. Precipitating factors include infection, myocardial
   infarction, stroke, trauma or prolonged exposure to cold
   environment.

Clinical evaluation
1. Ask for increasing somnolensce, stupor, coma or fits.
2. Frequently past history of surgery or radioiodine treatment for thyrotoxicosis.
3. Weight gain, slowness, voice change and other symptoms of hypothyroidism.
4. A precipitating cause such as exposure to cold weather,
   infection, trauma, stroke etc.
5. Clinical examination: temperature (hypothermia), mental
   status, HR (severe bardycardia), hypoventilation, goitre,
   hyporeflexia, dry, cold and coarse skin and if conscious,
   a hoarse or brassy voice.
6. Look for heart failure.
7. Exclude a hypopituitary state.

Investigations
1. FBC, electrolytes, urea and creatinine, ABG, free thyroxine and TSH levels.
2. ECG.

3. CXR.
4. Tests to exclude suspected precipitating cause(s).
5. Tests to exclude hypopituitarism, if indicated.

Management

1. IV T3 (triiodothyronine) 5–20 μg slowly q12 hours: caution if ischaemic heart disease present. If IV T3 is not available, IV T4 may be used (IV T4 : 12.5–50 ug 12 hourly).
2. IV hydrocortisone 100 mg 8 hourly (important especially if hypo-pituitary state suspected).
3. Treat hypothermia with warm blankets in warm room.
4. High flow oxygen if cyanosis is present.
5. Treat complications such as hypoglycaemia, heart failure etc.
6. Treat precipitating cause(s).

ADRENAL INSUFFICIENCY
LEE KOK ONN

Adrenal insufficiency is important primarily for the deficiency of the glucocorticoid, cortisol, with or without a concommitant deficiency in the mineralocorticoid, aldosterone.

Causes
1. Primary —Involvement of the adrenal glands in infection (TB, histoplasmosis), autoimmune disease, or acute haemorrhagic infarction (sepsis or DIVC). Both cortisol and aldosterone are low, and ACTH is elevated.
2. Secondary from deficiency of ACTH. Commoner causes are post-cranial or nasopharynx irradiation and acute withdrawal of steroid therapy (including those found in traditional medical preparations). Sheehan's syndrome is rarely seen in Singapore now. Only cortisol is low.

Clinical evaluation
1. A high index of suspicion is important as symptoms and signs are non-specific, mortality is significant and treatment with cortisol is easy and life-saving.
2. Suspicious symptoms include fatigue, weight loss without an obvious reason, symptoms of postural hypotension. A history of cranial irradiation, infection, or other autoimmune disease may be present.
3. Suggestive findings include hypotension, hyponatraemia, hypoglycaemia, especially if any of these are present in a patient with obvious signs of Cushing's syndrome. Otherwise the patient is usually thin.
4. Sudden development of hypotensive shock, hyponatraemia and hypoglycaemia, in an ill patient with a suspicious history. An adrenal crisis may be triggered in susceptible patients by mild illness, infection, trauma or surgery.

Investigations

1. Electrolytes, urea and creatinine, cortisol and ACTH levels.
2. Imaging as dictated by suspected cause: AXR for calcification of adrenal glands, CT head scan for assessing pituitary fossa.

Management

1. In an emergency, where the patient is acutely ill, the response to IV hydrocortisone 100 mg twice daily is sufficient evidence while awaiting blood results. If hypotension and hyponatraemia are corrected by this dose of hydrocortisone, a presumptive diagnosis of adrenal insufficiency can be made, and the patient should be maintained on IV hydrocortisone at the same dose.
2. Definitive diagnosis is best left to an endocrinologist. It is safest to keep the patient on near physiological replacement doses of hydrocortisone until a clear diagnosis is made. Oral hydrocortisone 20 mg in the morning, and 10 mg in the evening is a commonly used regime, with instructions to the patient to double the dose if there is stress e.g. infection, injury, etc.

HYPERCALCAEMIA
CHIONH SIOK BEE

Diagnosis based on both raised adjusted total and ionised calcium levels.

Adjusted total Calcium = total calcium + (40 − serum albumin) × 0.02 mmol/l.

Clinical evaluation
1. Symptoms non-specific, include anorexia, nausea, constipation, thirst, polyuria, weakness, malaise, confusion, obtundation and nephrolithiasis.
2. Look for clinical clues for the cause of hypercalcaemia: common causes — malignancy, primary hyperparathyroidism, drugs, e.g. $CaCO_3$, calcitriol; common precipitating factors — dehydration, immobilisation, thiazide treatment.
3. Assess degree of volume depletion and complicating factors (e.g. renal failure).

Investigations
1. Electrolytes, urea and creatinine, total calcium and inoised calcium, serum albumin, PTH.
2. 24-hour urine calcium.
3. ECG.
4. CXR, KUB.

Management
1. For severe hypercalcaemia (total calcium > 3.3 mmol/l):
   (i)   Stop drugs contributing to hypercalcaemia — $CaCO_3$, calcitriol, 1 (-calcidol, thiazides,
   (ii) Rehydrate with IV normal saline 2.5–4 litres/day,
   (iii) When patient adequately hydrated, give IV frusemide 10–20 mg 6 hourly,
   (iv) Give IV biphosphonate (contraindicated in significant renal failure) OR calcitonin (more rapid onset) as follows: IV clodronate 5 mg/kg in 500 ml normal

saline over 4 hours daily for 3–5 days OR IV pamidronate 30–90 mg over 4 hours × 1 dose (30 mg in mild renal failure); IV Calcitonin 4–8 IU/kg (usually 100–200 units) 8–12 hourly.

(v) For haematological malignancies (lymphoma, myeloma), and vitamin D excess states (e.g. sarcoidosis), give IV hydrocortisone 100 mg 8 hourly × 3–5 days OR oral prednisolone 20 mg 8 hourly.

(vi) Check serum K^+ and Ca^{2+} 4 hourly, replace K^+ as necessary.

(vii) Treat underlying cause for hypercalcaemia.

2. For moderate hypercalcaemia (total calcium 2.8–3.3 mmol/l): therapy depends on severity of symptoms, generally the same as for severe hypercalcaemia but need not be as aggressive (hydration and frusemide may be sufficient).

3. For mild hypercalcaemia (total calcium 2.5–2.8 mmol/l):

(i) Stop drugs contributing to hypercalcaemia,

(ii) Hydrate orally and ambulate,

(iii) Treat underlying cause.

HEMATOLOGY/ONCOLOGY

BLEEDING DISORDERS
LIU TE CHIH and KUPERAN P

Introduction
Usual presentation is spontaneous bleeding.
Ecchymoses indicate a clotting or platelet disorder.
Petechiae indicate a platelet disorder (thrombocytopenia or platelet dysfunction).

Clinical evaluation
1. Common causes: thrombocytopaenia, DIC, liver disease, over-anticoagulation; haemophilia/acquired factor VIII inhibitor.
2. Check for features of shock (hypotension, tachycardia, mental obtundation, reduced urine output) or significant hypovolaemia (postural hypotension, tachycardia, cool peripheries).
3. Is it a dangerous bleed?
   (i) Potentially life-threatening — gastrointestinal, intracranial bleeds;
   (ii) Moderately dangerous — head and neck bleed, compartment syndrome, retroperitoneal or ilio-psoas bleed, haematuria;
   (iii) Not so dangerous — joint, skin bleeding.
4. What is the cause for bleeding disorder?
   (i) Sick patient — severe infections, liver disease, DIC;
   (ii) Purpura/mucosal bleeding — thrombocytopaenia;
   (iii) Large ecchymoses, haematoma — coagulation factor defects.
   Bleeding in DIC usually occurs only when platelets are low, and/or fibrinogen is low. When there is only 1 haemostatic defect, e.g. isolated thrombocytopenia or raised PTT, there is usually no spontaneous bleeding.

Investigations
FBC, PT/PTT/TCT, ± blood group and cross-match. If isolated prolonged APTT, ask for correction with normal plasma.

Management

1. IV fluid resuscitation for shock or hypovolaemia.
2. Stop bleeding with local measures where applicable.
3. Correct bleeding disorder:
    (i) Clotting abnormalities: The need for clotting factor replacement is determined clinically. Lab tests are a guide at best. In the presence of bleeding, a PT/PTT persistently $> 1.5 \times$ mean normal clotting time or a fibrinogen level < 1 g/L usually indicates a need for correction.

    Fresh Frozen Plasma (FFP) –10 ml/kg initial dose and 500 ml 8 hourly. Usually a temporary measure as volume load to patient is large;

    Cryoprecipitate — rich in Factor VIII and fibrinogen; usual dose of 10 bags sufficient to raise fibrinogen to haemostatic levels;

    Factor VIII concentrate — usually for treatment of haemophilia, dose = [target level $\times$ body wt (kg) $\times$ 0.5] twice daily, aim for target trough VIII levels of 30%, 50% and 75% for mild, moderate and severe bleeds respectively; Factor IX concentrate — dose = [target level $\times$ body wt (kg)] once daily, target levels as for Factor VIII.

    (ii) Thrombocytopenia — Decision about platelet transfusion: presence of clinical features is more important than the absolute platelet count — febrile, associated coagulation abnormalities, site of bleeding, and interventional procedures. Consider platelet transfusion prophylactically if platelets $< 20 \times 10^9$/L, with intraocular/intracranial bleeding if with platelet level $< 100 \times 10^9$/L; with gastrointestinal bleed if platelets $< 80 \times 10^9$/L.

    Random platelets — usual dose is 6 units or 1 bag per 10 kg body weight. Each unit can be expected to increase patient's platelet count by 5 – 10×10^9/L.

    Apheresed platelets — collected by prior arrangement with Blood donation centre. Each bag equivalent to 6 units of random platelets.

ANTICOAGULATION
LIU TE CHIH and KUPERAN P

Introduction

Anticoagulation is usually indicated for treatment of deep vein thrombosis ± pulmonary embolism, for prosthetic cardiac valves and for atrial fibrillation and cardiac conditions which predispose to thromboembolism (e.g. dilated cardiomyopathy).

Long-term anticoagulation is usually achieved with oral warfarin.

Unreliable or mentally subnormal patients are not good candidates for oral anticoagulation therapy. Low molecular weight heparin would be a safer alternative in such cases.

Contraindications to anticoagulation

1. Haemorrhagic CVA.
2. Known peptic ulcer disease.
3. Known bleeding diathesis.
4. Recent neurosurgery.

Anticoagulation with conventional heparin and oral warfarin

See Figure.

Low molecular weight heparin (LMWH)

1. No monitoring is generally required for therapy with LMWH.
2. The pharmacokinetics may be different in certain situations and monitoring assays for LMWH may be advisable in children, obese individuals and in renal failure.
3. Dosing for therapeutic anticoagulation with Fraxiparine™
   Body weight up to 50 kg: 0.5 ml bd
   Body weight 51–60 kg: 0.6 ml bd
   Body weight 61–70 kg: 0.7 ml bd
   Dosing for prophylaxis is similar but at once a day.

(Dosing is different for other makes of LMWH. If a different supplier of LMWH is used, follow the manufacturer's recommended doses.)

Reversal of oral anticoagulation

1. Life-threatening haemorrhage: IV Vitamin K 5 mg, and Fresh Frozen Plasma (FFP) 10 ml/kg initial dose and repeat if INR still excessively high; may consider Factor IX (prothrombin complex) 50 U/kg.
2. Less severe haemorrhage: IV Vitamin K 0.5–1 mg, and stop warfarin for 2 days, then review.
3. INR > 4.5 without bleeding — stop warfarin for 2 days, then review.
4. Unexpected bleeding at therapeutic levels — look for a secondary cause for the bleeding.

NOTES:
1. Doses may have to adjusted downwards for smaller or debilitated patients.
2. Indians on average require a higher dose to achieve an equivalent level of anticoagulation.
3. Monitoring of warfarin therapy shouold be closer if patient is on a number of other drugs (e.g. antibiotics, cimetidine, etc) as fluctuations from interactions are likely.

COMMON MEDICAL PROBLEMS IN CANCER PATIENTS

JOHN WONG

Neutropenic Fever

This is an emergency. Suspect in all patients on chemotherapy with temperature greater than 38°C.

Definition

Temperature greater than 38°C when the absolute neutrophil count (ANC) is less than 1000. The ANC is calculated by mutiplying the percent neutrophils by the total white cell count, e.g. neutrophils 30%, total white cell 3,000 : ANC = 900.

Clinical evaluation

1. Wash your hands.
2. Check oral temperature, pulse rate, blood pressure, and respiratory rate.
3. Any known drug allergies?
4. Practice strict asepsis in all procedures, especially blood drawing, insertion of IV lines.
5. Examine for skin lesions, sinus tenderness, oropharyngeal lesions, including dental infections, pneumonia, intra-abdominal source, check the perianal area.
6. No rectal and vaginal examinations unless ordered by the oncologist.

Investigations

1. FBC with differential count, electrolytes, urea and creatinine, liver function tests.
2. Septic workup: blood cultures × 2 (one from each arm), urine for FEME and culture, sputum culture if available, culture any purulent discharge.
3. CXR.

Management

1. Antibiotics (assuming no penicillin allergy) — to be given IV after blood cultures:
   (i) IV ceftazidime 1.0 to 2.0 grams q8hrs.
   (ii) If obvious skin source, add IV cloxacillin 1 G q6hrs. If penicillin allergic, consider IV ciprofloxacin 200 mg q12hrs, IV gentamicin (vide infra). If skin source seen, add IV clindamycin 600 mg q8hrs.
2. Trace the full blood count after 1 hour. Calculate the absolute neutrophil count (ANC).
3. If the patient looks unwell, and/or if ANC is less than 500, add IV gentamicin 2 mg/kg load, followed by 1.5 mg/kg every 8 hours. Check a trough level after 3 doses.
4. Trace the renal function 4 hours after sending the specimen and consider adjusting your antibiotic dosing schedule if evidence of renal insufficiency.
5. Trace blood cultures and adjust antibiotics accordingly.
6. Wash hands before entering patient's room.
7. No intramuscular injections (IM)
8. Change all intravenous sites every 3 days
9. If possible, nurse the patient in a single room. If that is not possible, attempt to have non-infectious patients in the same cubicle.
10. No urinary catheters

Cord Compression

This is one of the worst things to happen to a cancer patient, and should not be allowed to develop if at all possible. This is an emergency. Suspect in any cancer patient who complains of back pain. Do not wait for weakness, sensory changes, or decreased reflexes to develop, as it may be too late by then.

Definition

Compression of the spinal cord by tumor.

Clinical evaluation
1. Where is the back pain?
2. Any change in sensation or strength?
3. Press each spinous process.
4. Careful evaluation of muscle strength, sensation, and reflexes.

Investigations
1. Urgent plain spine X-rays first, PA and lateral.
2. If the plain X-ray is normal, decide whether to screen with a bone scan first, or proceed to a non-urgent MRI.
3. MRI.

Management
1. Known History of Cancer (Pathology Established):
   (i)   If vertebra collapsed, or pedicle absent on plain X-rays, start IV dexamethasone 16 mg in 50 mls normal saline infusion immediately, followed by 4 mg slow bolus every 6 hours. Arrange an urgent MRI.
   (ii) If cord compression is strongly suspected or confirmed, start IV dexamethasone.
   (iii) Prophylax for oral candidiasis with oral nystatin 500,000 units tds.
   (iv) Watch blood sugar.
   (v)   Refer for urgent radiotherapy once MRI confirms level.
2. No Known History of Cancer — Urgent orthopedic surgical consultation for tissue diagnosis as well as decompression. Note that the majority of compression is anterior and needs anterior decompression rather than posterior laminectomy.

Hypercalcemia of malignancy
This a common problem and difficult to diagnose as symptoms and signs are non-specific. Suspect in all cancer patients who don't feel well, especially in cancers associated with hypercalcemia, e.g. squamous cell, breast, lymphomas, myelomas, clear cell. If untreated, this can be life-threatening.

Definition
Elevated ionised calcium. If your laboratory only reports total calcium, you need to correct if the albumin is low.

Clinical evaluation
1. Symptoms and signs range from aches and pain, to constipation, lethargy, thirst, polyuria, confusion, and obtundation.
2. Look for dehydration, e.g. tissue turgor, tongue, postural tachycardia, postural hypotension.

Investigations
1. Serum ionised calcium (or total calcium and albumin), electrolytes, urea and creatinine.

Management
1. Aggressive hydration with IV normal saline; may need up to 3–4 litres in the first 24 hours in severe cases.
2. Save diuretics only for impending fluid overload as premature use may make hypercalcemia worse.
3. Start IV clodronate 300 mg in 500 mls normal saline over 3 hours after the patient is adequately hydrated; repeat daily for 3 to 5 days.
4. Consider prednisone if patient has breast cancer, myeloma, or lymphoma.
5. Start oral clodronate once hypercalcemia under control.

RHEUMATOLOGICAL EMERGENCIES

NG SWEE CHENG

Emergencies in Systemic Lupus Erythematosus (SLE)

The febrile SLE patient

1. Main clinical decision is whether the fever is due to active SLE, infection or both.

Favouring active SLE	Favouring infection
Clinical signs of activity e.g. alopecia, malar or photosensitive rash, oral ulcers, cutaneous vasculitis, polyarthritis, serositis	Focus of infection e.g. purulent sputum suggesting pneumonia, dysuria suggesting urinary tract infection
History of precipitating event e.g. stress, non-compliance with medication	History of exposure to infection e.g. TB
White cell count often low; Hb and platelets may be low	White cell count high; Hb and platelets often normal
CRP normal; C3, C4 low, dsDNA high	CRP high; C3, C4 normal; dsDNA normal
Urinalysis dysmorphic RBCs, active urine sediment, proteinuria	Urinalysis: normal or pyuria with positive urine culture

2. Patients with active SLE should also be given antibiotics if there is the slightest suggestion of infection.
3. For SLE patients with infection, continue their usual dose of steroids and taper steroid dose when patient is stable.

Management

1. IV hydrocortisone 100 mg 6 hourly OR.

2. If patient is very ill or there is major target organ involvement, IV methylprednisolone 0.5–1 g om (over 30 minutes) for 3 days.
3. Consult senior doctor about use of cyclophosphamide or plasmapheresis.

SLE with major target organ involvement

Central nervous system (CNS) lupus
1. Clinical features: coma, psychosis, focal neurogical deficit, fits, movement disorders.
2. Differential diagnoses:
   (i)   Infections: brain abscess, TB meningitis,
   (ii) Drug overdosage in depressed SLE patients; steroid psychosis,
   (iii) Hypertensive encephalopathy,
   (iv) Metabolic problems: electrolyte imbalances, renal failure, diabetic emergencies,
   (v)   Cerebral infarction (accelerated atherosclerosis or anti-phospholipid syndrome),
   (vi) Cerebral haemorrhage from immune thrombocytopenia,
   (vii) Unrelated conditions e.g. schizophrenia, epilepsy,
3. Treatment: High dose steroids; consider anti-psychotic drugs as indicated.

Emergencies in Scleroderma

Scleroderma renal crisis

Severe hypertension with diastolic BP > 110 mm Hg plus 2 of the following:

- Hypertensive retinopathy > Grade II
- Proteinuria
- Azotaemia
- Microangiopathic haemolytic anaemia
- Seizures
- Haematuria
- Rapidly deteriorating renal function

Management

1. Start captopril 25 mg tds or enalapril 10 mg om and titrate dose to control BP.
2. If ACE inhibitors not tolerated, use calcium channel blockers e.g. felodipine
3. Give frusemide if fluid overload present
4. If severe acute renal failure develops, dialysis is required. Continue ACE inhibitors.

Raynaud's phenomenon

Attacks when cold with colour change from white to blue to red. When severe, can lead to gangrene of affected digits.

Management

1. Keep patient and extremities warm (avoid air-conditioning, wear gloves and socks).
2. Discontinue drugs which may aggravate vasospasm e.g. β-blockers.
3. Give aspirin 100 mg om.
4. In mild cases, give calcium channel blockers, e.g. nifedepine 10 mg tds or α-blockers e.g. prazosin 1 mg test dose, gradually increased to 2-5 mg tds if tolerated (watch BP).
5. In severe cases with impending gangrene: infusion of prostaglandin Ei via central venous line starting at 0.1 μg/kg/min to maximum 0.4 μg/kg/min, or; prostacyclin (or its analogue Iloprost), or infusion of pentoxifylline 100 mg/hour (maximum 1200 mg /day).
6. Give antibiotics if secondary infection of ischaemic ulcers is present
7. Avoid steroids and cytotoxic agents as Raynaud's is not due to vasculitis and as these agents increase the risk of secondary infection. Use these drugs only when vasculitis cannot be excluded particularly in patients with Overlap syndrome.

Emergencies in Rheumatoid Arthritis

Rheumatoid vasculitis
Usually seen in long standing sero-positive erosive RA or Felty's syndrome.

1. Mild localised stable vasculitis (e.g. nail fold infarcts, peripheral neuropathy):
   (i)   Low dose steroids, start with < 30 mg prednisolone daily,
   (ii) Disease modifying anti-rheumatic drugs, e.g. D-penicillamine, methotrexate,
   (iii) An NSAID to reduce inflammation and inhibit platelet function.

2. Systemic vasculitis (e.g. mononeuritis multiplex, digital infarcts, visceral involvement):
   (i)   High dose steroids (IV hydrocortisone or methyl-prednisolone),
   (ii) Cytotoxics e.g. cyclophosphamide 50 mg daily p.o.

3. Refractory vasculitis — IV immunoglobulins by infusion

C1–C2 subluxation
Usually seen in long standing sero-positive RA; also seen in other inflammatory arthrits e.g. spondyloarthropathy and psoriatic arthritis.

Clinical evaluation
1. Pain in occiput from C1 root irritation.
2. Weakness from cord compression.
3. Posterior cerebral symptoms from vertebral artery kinking.
4. Cervical spinal X-rays — best done under supervision by orthopaedic surgeon.

Management
1. Immobilise cervical spine with collar or cervical traction while MRI or CT myelogram is being arranged.

2. Urgent referral to orthopaedic surgeon.
3. Treat inflammatory synovitis with an NSAID and disease-modifying anti-rheumatic agent.

Acute Monoarthritis

Causes
1. Infection i.e. septic arthritis — Gonococcus, Staphylo-coccus.
2. Crystals — gout, calcium pyrophosphate.
3. Seronegative spondyloarthropathy — Reiter's syndrome, psoriatic arthritis.
4. Trauma.
5. Osteoarthritis.

Investigations
1. FBC, ESR, electrolytes, urea and creatinine, uric acid, RA factor.
2. X-ray of joint for erosions and joint destruction.
3. If infection suspected, culture blood and aspirate joint — send synovial fluid for Gram stain, polarising microscopy for urate crystals, bacterial culture.

Management
1. Start empirical antibiotic according to Gram stain result:
   (i)   Gram positive (Staphylococcus, Streptococcus) — IV cloxacillin; IV vancomycin if MRSA suspected.
   (ii) Gram negative cocci (Gonococcus) — IV Ceftriaxone 2 g daily
   (iii) Gram negative bacilli (Enterobacteriaceae, Pseudo-monas aeruginosa) — IV Ceftriaxone 1–2 g daily or IV Ceftazidime 1 g bd.
   (iv) Gram stain negative result: — give IV Ceftriaxone
2. Change antibiotics when culture results available.

Management of gout
1. Give an NSAID e.g. IM Diclofenac (Volteran) 50 mg or oral Indomethacin 50 mg tds OR oral colchicine 0.5 mg

hourly till improvement or side-effects (gastrointestinal complaints) or maximum dose of 4 mg/day, then continue colchicine 0.5 mg om.

2. Avoid NSAIDs if renal impairment or past or current history of peptic ulcer disease or gastrointestinal bleeding.

3. If neither NSAIDs or colchicine can be used, then give either:

    (i) Prednisolone 10 mg tds p.o. or IV hydrocortisone 100 mg stat, OR

    (ii) Analgesics e.g. IM Pethidine 50 mg stat.

4. Do not start allopurinol during acute gout as attack may get worse.

ICU

MECHANICAL VENTILATOR: FRIEND OR FOE
LEE KANG HOE

The mechanical ventilator provides positive pressure ventilation, and are usually volume-cycled. Mechanical ventilation
requires intubation which can be oro-tracheal or naso-tra-
cheal. Choose the biggest endotracheal tube the patient can
tolerate (female: 6.5 to 8.0, male: 7.5 to 9.0). Airway resistance increases as ETT size decreases. Bronchoscopy should
be performed with a minimum ETT size of 7.5.

Indications for mechanical ventilation (friend)
Important to document the reason for intubation and the
intubation process itself.
1. Acute respiratory failure — type I or type II.
2. Airway protection — e.g. gag absent, massive hema-
   temesis, intracranial pathology, intoxications.
3. Hyperventilation — severe acidosis.
4. Shock — reduce work of breathing to reduce proportion
   of cardiac output to respiratory muscles.

Problems associated with mechanical ventilation (Foe)
1. Barotrauma/volutrauma (alveolar overdistension) —
   pneumothorax, capillary leak.
2. Oxygen toxicity (keep FiO_2 < 60%).
3. Hypotension from decreased venous return.
4. Nosocomial pneumonia.
5. Morbidity or mortality from intubation.

Setting the ventilator:
1. Ensure that the oxygen and air connections are in place.
2. Turn on the ventilator.
3. Always start with a FiO_2 of 100% until a reading can
   be obtained on the pulse oximetry.
4. Choose the mode (start with AC* or SIMV + PS).
5. Set the tidal volume (6 to 9 ml/kg).

6. Set the rate (12 to 20 bpm) — if spontaneously breathing adjust to at least 80% of total rate.
7. Determine the I:E ratio — usually 1:2 (Adjust peak flow or set % insp time and % pause time).
8. Set PEEP — usually start at 5 cmH$_2$O.
9. Set sensitivity to –2 cmH$_2$O.
10. If PS mode employed, set at 15 to 20 cmH$_2$O
11. Adjust the appropriate alarms.

*AC vs. CMV or VC on most ventilators. The difference is the trigger sensitivity. If the patient can triggger a machine breath, it is AC mode. Thus, every inspiratory effort the patient makes will be machine assisted. If there are no spontaneous breaths, the machine will provide the set rate and tidal volume. Thus, AC can be used for patients who are not paralysed.

Evaluation
1. Check peak airway pressure — try to keep < 35 cmH$_2$O.
2. Keep oxygen stauration > 92% or PaO$_2$ > 60 mmHg.
3. Check ABG within 30 minutes — do not overventilate unless for raised ICP.
4. Check with the patient whether they feel comfortable.
5. Consider sedation (midazolam 1 to 5 mg/hr or propofol 100 to 400 mg/hr) and then paralysis (atracurium 0.5 mg/kg/hr), if the patient is "fighting" the ventilator or RR > 35 bpm.
6. Wean FiO$_2$ to < 0.6 using the pulse oximeter.
7. If peak airway pressure is high, allow for hypercapnia, assuming there is no raised ICP or significant hypotension.

Other important points
1. Mean airway pressure is linearly related to O$_2$ saturation.
2. Peak airway pressure does not reflect transalveolar pressure if airway resistance is high, e.g. asthma.
3. Pressure-controlled ventilation will provide a variable tidal volume depending on the compliance. It guarantees the peak airway pressure, and is easy to invert the I:E ratio.

4. Increasing PEEP will increase FRC and decrease shunt. High PEEP may however reduce cardiac output.
5. High peak airway pressures may indicate bronchospasm, pneumothorax, or a kinked tube. A high plateau pressure indicates a worsening of lung parenchymal disease.
6. In acute asthmatics, allow sufficient expiratory time — othersie autoPEEP will develop.
7. Try prone position for patients that have refractory hypoxemia.

INVASIVE HEMODYNAMIC MONITORING
LEE KANG HOE

Hemodynamic monitoring involves the measurement of heart-rate, blood pressure, any other central pressures (RA, PA, PAWP), and flow measurements (cardiac output).

Non-invasive methods should be considered first before invasive methods are employed because of the higher morbidity associated with invasive methods.

Blood pressure
Indications for Intra-arterial lines:
  (i) close monitoring of the blood pressure is required (unstable patient, titration of vasoactive substances)
  (ii) frequent arterial blood gas determinations.

Sites: radial artery (commonest site, ensure good ulnar collateral circulation). Other sites are the dorsal pedalis, femoral, axillary and brachial (this is an end-artery).

Check that the transducer is appropriately zeroed and level for the reading.

Watch the waveform — the systolic pressure may be falsely elevated. Verify with the cuff pressure (note when the arterial pulse returns). The mean arterial pressure from the femoral artery is the closest approximation to central aortic pressure.

Central lines
Indications:
  (i) Venous access, especially for large catheters for dialysis or large volume infusions.
  (ii) Measurement of RA pressure (estimate of pre-load — but notoriously inaccurate especially with water manometers, and in the setting of pulmonary hypertension).

Sites: internal jugular veins, subclavian veins, or even occasionally, the external jugular vein.

Measurement: take the nadir for patients on positive-pressure ventilation and the peak for those breathing spontaneously.

Pulmonary artery catheters
Indications:
   (i)   Measure PAWP as an estimate of pre-load.
   (ii)   Determination of cardiac output.
   (iii) Measurement of mixed venous oxygen saturation.
   (iv)   Also allows measurement of RA, RV, and PA pressures.

Important to have the above information when patient is on high-dose inotropes, severe ARDS, or in renal failure where there is a question of pre-renal cause. Pt has to be in ICU. Sites: internal jugular veins, subclavian veins, femoral veins. Balloon-flotation catheter positioned at the bedside by following the changes in pressure waveform (figure 1). Occasionally, fluoroscopy is required to help obtain placement. PAWP is assumed to reflect LV pressures assuming there is no mitral valve disease, and that LV pressure reflects LV volumes which determines preload according to Starling's law. However, if the LV compliance is altered, e.g. ischemia, then the pressure measurement may not accurately reflect LV volumes. In order to measure PAWP, the tip has to be in zone III (West's). Otherwise, alveolar pressures can also affect PAWP measurement. A "pop-off" PAWP will eliminate this effect.

Patient in shock:
   (i)   Ensure PAWP is 15 to 18 mmHg (titrate to maximal CI),
   (ii)   Optimise CI > 4.5 L/min/m^2 (inotropes required),
   (iii) Keep SvO$_2$ > 60%.
(Do not use SVR to titrate vasopressors, as SVR may be low when there are areas of vasocontriction, as the SVR reflects the total resistance which is the reciprocal.)
Patient with ARDS:
   (i)   Keep PAWP between 10 to 12 mmHg,
   (ii)   Ensure adequate CI > 4.5 L/min/m^2.

Complications:
1. All invasive catheters: Infection, thrombosis, aneurysm, bleeding.

2. CVP and PA catheters: pneumothorax, arrhthymias.
3. PA catheters: pulmonary artery rupture.

Dampened PA waveform:
1. Flush the catheter — exclude any air bubbles in the line.
2. Check that the connections are tight.
3. Pull the catheter out until the PA waveform is present again.

Performing a cardiac output:
1. Ensure that the cardiac output computer is connected.
2. Key in the height and weight of the patient.
3. Check that the computational constant for that particular PA catheter is correctly keyed-in.
4. Check that the external temperature probe is placed correctly in a plastic ampoule of water at room temperature.
5. Inject 10 cc of water as fast as possible through the RA port.
6. Perform a minimum of 3 measurements — preferable 5.
7. Record the pressure measurements and the inotropes present.

Calculated variables
1. SVRI (dynes.sec/cm^{5}M^2) = ({MAP – CVP} $\times$ 80)/CI
2. PVRI = ({PAP – PAWP} $\times$ 80)/CI
3. Oxygen delivery (DO$_2$) = CI $\times$ CaO$_2$
4. CaO$_2$ (vol%) = (1.3 $\times$ Hb $\times$ SaO$_2$) + (0.003 $\times$ PaO$_2$)

Interpretation
Cardiac output should be interpretated with the following information: inotropes, heart rate, PAWP, MAP, lactate, acid-base status, urine output and patient's overall status. It is important to repeat the measurements over time to monitor the trend. Cardiac output is adequate if the end-organs are receiving adequate perfusion according to demands.

Septic patients: commonly has high CI (> 4.0 L/min/m^2), with a lowish PAWP and a high lactate.
Cardiogenic shock: commonly low CI (< 2.5 L/min/m^2) with a high PAWP.
Pulmonary embolism: low CI, low PAWP, high PA and RV pressures.

Abbreviations

CaO$_2$ — arterial oxygen content
CO — cardiac output
CI — cardiac index

CVP — central venous pressure

DO$_2$ — oxygen delivery
Hb — hemoglobin
MAP — mean arterial pressure

PA — pulmonary artery
PaO$_2$ — partial pressure of oxygen
PAWP — pulmonary artery wedge pressure
PVRI — pulmonary vascular resistance index
RA — right atrium
SaO$_2$ — arterial oxygen saturation
SVRI — systemic vascular resistance index

MISCELLANEOUS

POISONING
LEE KANG HOE

General principles

Even if there is no clear history of poisoning, consider the possibility for all confused and comatose patients. Perform drug levels on all the common drugs (paracetamol, salicylate, benzodiazepine, tricyclic antidepressants, opioids, ethanol) besides the drug supposedly ingested — multiple drug ingestions are common. Establish suicide risk.

Assessment and management

1. History — obtain information on drug/toxin ingested (how much, when, and route).
2. Physical — establish ABCs, neurological status (pupils) and airway protection, vital signs.
3. Investigations:
   (a) Laboratory: FBC, SP#1, Hypocount, drug levels/ toxicology, ABG (look out for metabolic acidosis, especially high anion gap)
   (b) ECG
   (c) Chest radiograph as indicated.
4. IV access x 2.
5. Oxygen supplementation.
6. In comatose patients, consider the following antidotes: glucose 50% (50 mL iv), thiamine (100 mg), flumazenil (Anexate, 0.2–3 mg iv), and naloxone (Narcan, 0.4–2 mg iv) for comatose patients. Beware of seizures with flumazenil in tricyclic overdoses. Give medication one by one and document the effect of each drug.
7. Gastric lavage (contraindicated in strong acid or alkali ingestions) with activated charcoal (50G). Intubate patient if gag is absent before the lavage.
8. Consider antidote as appropriate or forced alkaline diuresis (salicylic acid, phenobarbital, chlorpropamide).
9. Admit to ICU if ECG abnormalities, hemodynamic instability, airway management problem, or requires hemo-

dialysis (severe ethylene glycol, lithium, methanol, and salicylate poisonings) or charcoal hemoperfusion (theophylline, barbiturates).

10. If severe acidosis, exclude DKA and check levels of lactate, but beware of salicylate, ethanol and methanol (look for osmolar gap).

Specific drug overdoses

1. Paracetamol overdose — Obtain 4 hour serum level. Give N-acetylcysteine in all cases of paracetamol overdose (do not wait for levels) — 150 mg/kg in 200 mL 5% dextrose over 30 min, then 50 mg/kg in 500 ml 5% dextrose over 4 hr, and then the same over next 8 hr, and again in the next 8 hrs. Anaphylaxis is rare.

2. Insecticide poisoning (cholinesterase inhibitors) — Remove exposure (e.g. contaminated clothes). Muscarinic: salivation, lacrimation, urination, defaecation, gastrointestinal distress, and emesis (SLUDGE). Nicotinic: muscle fasciculations, cramping, weakness, hypertension, tachycardia, and pupillary dilation. Give atropine (2 to 4 mg iv) for muscarinic symptoms — repeat every 30 minutes as needed, up to 100 mg until relieve of muscarinic symptoms. Give IV pralidoxime (PAM) 1G q4 hrs for 24 to 48 hours.

3. Tricyclic antidepressants — main problem is arrhythmia (treat with bicarbonate — keep pH between 7.45 to 7.5, as first line before other anti-arrhythmics). Other symptoms are part of the anticholinergic syndrome (hyperthermia, dry, red, confusion, urinary retention, and mydriasis). More severely, they may have hypotension and seizures, plus coma without brain-stem reflexes. Do not giver physostigmine — risk of exacerbating conduction blockade or seizure.

4. Opioids — naloxone is a specific antagonist. Usually given as 0.01 mg/kg — higher doses may be required. If respiratory depression present, give 2 mg iv stat. Lasts approximately 20 to 60 minutes. May require repeat dosing (0.4 to 4 mg/hr).

5. Barbiturates — alkaline diuresis (only effective for phe-nobarbitone and not the shorter acting barbiturates): give a bolus of 100 ml 8.4% sodium bicarbonate, followed by a continuous infusion of 500 ml D5% with 50 mL of 8.4% sodium bicarbonate plus 25 mmol KCl, at a rate of 150 ml/hour. Watch for fluid overload and hypokalaemia. Keep urine pH 7.5 to 8.
6. Salicylates — symptoms of tinnitus, deafness, nausea, vomiting, tremor, sweating, hyperventilation, agitation, confusion. If > 4.3 mmol/L or has manifestations of salicylism, consider forced alkaline diuresis. If severe acidosis, altered mental status, or very high levels, con-sider hemodialysis.

ADVERSE DRUG REACTIONS
VERNON OH

Adverse drug reactions (ADRs) are unwanted effects of drugs. Due to either toxic or side-effects.
1) Toxic effect — exaggeration of the pharmacological action that produces the therapeutic effect of the drug,
2) Side-effect — occurs through another pharmacological action than that which produces the therapeutic effect, e.g. hypersensitivity reactions which are dose-independent and unpredictable.

The most serious acute ADR is an immediate hypersensitivity response (anaphylaxis) which ranges from "localised" forms such as urticaria, or angio-oedema, to "generalised" anaphylaxis (full-blown shock).

Management

Skin reaction
Irritating ADRs include toxic erythema and urticaria. Reassure the patient, and give a fast-acting antihistamine like acrivastine (adults, Semprex™ 8 mg tid) or cetirizine (children, 2.5–5 mg bid) followed by a sedating drug like chlorpheniramine or promethazine. If cutaneous reactions turn serious, e.g. erythema multiforme into Stevens-Johnson syndrome or toxic epidermal necrolysis, then refer the patient urgently to a dermatologist and the Burns Unit at Singapore General Hospital. Where the reaction was mild and the drug is potentially life-saving, e.g. antibiotic, consider referring patients for skin patch testing.

Airflow obstruction
Treat as for conventional acute asthma. However, you should observe the patient carefully and consider giving adrenaline when asthma occurs together with urticaria, angio-oedema or hypotension.

Angio-oedema
Mild attacks need intravenous promethazine 25–50 mg and may be followed by oral antihistamine. A 2–4 day course of oral prednisolone 20–40 mg, depending on body weight, decreases tissue swelling. Severe angio-oedema occurring together with wheeze may require intramuscular adrenaline 0.25–1.0 mg (0.25–1.0 ml of 1:1000 solution). Life-threatening angio-oedema (stridor or obvious breathing difficulty) may also require a surgical airway (cricothyroidotomy, or tracheostomy).

Anaphylactic shock
This emergency requires forethought for effective treatment. Anaphylactic shock can kill within minutes if untreated. Many patients experience extreme nausea, and an urge to pass urine and faeces, before confusion sets in. Central chest pain, breathlessness, and tachycardia often occur.

A management strategy should contain the following elements, which you may have to telescope together to save life:

Step 1: Basic life support: airway, breathing, circulation; reassure the patient;

Step 2: Correct cardiovascular collapse or severe systemic upset;

Step 3: Observe for 2–3 days;

Step 4: Remove the offending agent if practicable;

Step 5: Prevent recurrence.

Step 1
First secure an airway. You may need to intubate the patient for artificial ventilation. If anaphylaxis progresses rapidly, a surgical airway may be required. Having secured an airway, you should *raise the patient's legs* to help maintain the blood pressure, and *give high flow oxygen*. Set up two intravenous lines, one for infusion of isotonic saline and the other for injection of drugs. Repeatedly reassure the patient, who is likely to be terrified both by the discomfort of anaphylaxis and your treatment.

Step 2

Give adrenaline by intramuscular injection. If the patient is severely ill, inject adrenaline as a slow i.v. bolus injection. If venous access is difficult, waste no time in giving the drug i.m. In most adults the dose is 0.5–1.0 mg, choosing 0.5 mg for those weighing 50 kg and for mild anaphylaxis. Use the 1/1000 solution for i.m. injection, and *only* the 1/10 000 solution for slow i.v. injection (5–10 ml). Give promethazine 25–50 mg or diphenhydramine 10–50 mg as a slow i.v. bolus injection. You may start oral chlorpheniramine 6–12 mg 8 hourly as it acts slowly.

Give salbutamol by nebuliser for a mild reaction, and salbutamol 250 micrograms i.v. over 60 s, then 5–20 micrograms/min by infusion in severe airflow obstruction, or when the patient is taking a non-selective fl-blocker. Or use aminophylline 5mg/kg i.v. over 20 min, then 0.5 mg/hour.

Step 3

Monitor in MICU. Some patients relapse after some hours free of symptoms. Repeat the administration of adrenaline and bronchodilator as needed, until the blood pressure recovers. Persistent hypotension may require i.v. infusion of dopamine 5–20 micrograms/kg/min. Maintain antihistamine cover for 24–48 hours. In severely affected patients, you should give hydrocortisone 100 mg (5–10 mg in a child) i.v. over 60 s, and start oral prednisolone 0.5 mg/kg for 2–5 days. Corticosteroid helps prevent late relapses.

Step 4

Consider accelerating the clearance of the trigger drug (or substance) if it was taken in overdose or has a long half-time of elimination. Only some drugs are usefully removed by haemodialysis. Seek specialist advice from a clinical pharmacologist, pharmacist, or nephrologist.

Step 5

Prevent recurrence of anaphylaxis by first identifying the trigger substance. Flag the medical record clearly and check the tagging of the patient in the National Patient Master Index (MOH). Educate the patient and carer(s) to avoid the trigger. Medik Awas tagging is an option.

In severe allergy to insect stings or foods, e.g. peanuts, consider teaching the patient to use (when necessary) a prepared needle-syringe containing adrenaline 1.0 mg for self-injection i.m. or subcutaneously. Min-I-Jet, Epipen, or Ana-Guard syringes contain adrenaline 1/1000 solution.

NUTRITION
LEE KANG HOE

It is assumed that nutritional support is important for patients that are either malnourished or unable to maintain a normal diet in the face of illness. It is conventional to consider such supplementation after 3 days without food.

The preferred route is enteral for the following reasons: natural route, cheaper, less risk of infections, enterocytes derive their nutrition from the luminal contents, and decreased stress ulceration. If the enteral route cannot be employed, parenteral routes have to be considered: peripheral or central access.

The main concerns about enteral feeding are gastroparesis, aspiration and diarrhoea. Nursing the patient at 30^0 to the horizontal is the most effective way to prevent aspiration. Gastroparesis can be treated with motility agents like cisapride (10 mls tid NG) or metoclopromide (10 mg iv tid), or the placement of naso-enteric tubes. Diarrhoea may not be from the feeds (exclude antibiotic-induced and clostridium). Consider lower osmolality feeds with higher fibre.

The calorie requirements (non-protein) range from 30 to 35 kcal/kg/day. This is usually provided as a mixture of carbohydrates and lipids (60:40 to 40:60 ratios). The daily protein requirement is 1 to 1.5 G/kg (beware renal patients not on dialysis and liver failure patients). Take ideal body weight.

Feeds can be provided continuously or intermittently.

Enteral formulations available:

Formula	Calories (kcal/mL)	Protein (G/L)	Osmolality (mOsm/L)	Comments
Isocal*	1	34	270	isotonic
Ensure	1.06	37.2	470	low residue
Jevity	1.06	44	310	high fibre
Nepro	2	69.9	635	low K
Pulmocare	1.5	41	465	low CHO:fat

*Formulary in NUH

Pulmocare is purported to reduce CO_2 production but the evidence suggests that this is related to overfeeding rather than the CHO:fat ratio.

For example:
60 kg patient would require 1800 kcal and 60 G protein per day.
Isocal 1800 mL/day would provide 1800 kcal and 61.2 G protein.

If parenteral nutrition is required, a total parenteral form is required. Note that 500 mL of 5% dextrose provides only 100 kcal.

HEAT STROKE
R SURI

Introduction
In heat stroke, body temperature rises precipitously causing multisystem tissue damage and organ failure. Tissue injury is mediated by endotoxins, cytokines, activated coagulation components or injured endothelium. Classic heat stroke, affecting the aged and chronically ill, occurs mainly during heat waves, presents with hyperpyrexia, coma and hot, dry skin. Exertional heat stroke affects young, unacclimatized athletes or army recruits and usually presents with acute derangement of mental function, confusion, seizures or frank coma, with or without a prodrome.

Diagnostic Points
1. Hyperthermia: rectal temperature above 40°C.
2. Severe CNS disturbance: coma, delirium, convulsions, decerebrate posturing.
3. Hypotension: hypovolemia, myocardial damage, peripheral vasodilatation.
4. Hematological findings: DIVC, leucocytosis, normal or low platelets.
5. Biochemical abnormalities:
   (i) Early on, serum Na, K, Ca, PO_4 and Mg levels are frequently low.
   (ii) Classical HS: hyperglycaemia, hypophosphatemia, raised CK.
   (iii) Exertional HS: hyperkalemia, hyperphosphatemia and renal failure (oliguric). Rhabdomyolysis and hypocalcemia may occur.
   (iv) Hepatic damage (raised liver enzymes) in most patients (hepatic failure rare).
6. Mixed acid-base disorder: respiratory alkalosis with metabolic acidosis.
7. Sweating may or may not be present.
8. Hypoxaemia: lung injury (ARDS)

Differential Diagnosis

Heat stroke is sometimes a diagnosis of exclusion. The clinical diagnosis of heat stroke is strongly suggested when hyperthermia is associated with neurological dysfunction after exposure to high ambient temperature. Exclude: meningitis, encephalitis, intracranial hemorrhage, malaria, delirium tremens, thyrotoxic crisis, malignant hyperthermia, typhoid fever.

Investigations

1. FBC, electrolytes, urea and creatinine, LFT, DIC, calcicum, phosphate, ABG, lactate, CK, aldolase, X-match.
2. Urine for microscopy and myoglobin.
3. CXR.
4. ECG.

Management

1. First Aid (in the field) — Cooling measures should begin immediately as severity of the multisystem damage is related to the duration of hyperthermia. Remove patient to a cool, shady place. Loosen and remove clothing as is necessary. Splash tap water on patient and promote evaporation by fanning. Cold packs can be applied to axillae, groin and neck. Evacuate to a hospital as soon as possible ALL PATIENTS while continuing these measures.

2. Emergency Treatment (AandE) — ABCs'. IV access.

3. Continuous core temperature monitoring via a rectal thermometer.

4. Cooling should be intensified according to available resources if core temperature is still above 39°C (see below).

5. Consider admission to ICU.

6. Cooling — Despite cooling, about 25% of patients experience failure of one or more organ-systems. Rate of cooling should ideally be 0.1°C per minute with correction of hyperthermia in 45 to 60 mins. When core temperature falls to 38–39°C cooling should be stopped

to avoid shivering and a hypothermia overshoot. Core temperature monitoring should continue for at least 48–72 hrs as a rebound rise or temperature instability may persist.

(i) Body Cooling Unit (BCU) — An ideal cooling method using evaporative cooling. Patient is placed naked on a net surface facing finely atomised spray of water (15°C) and circulation of room air maintained by using portable electric fans.

(ii) Ice Water Bath Immersion — Although greater heat loss may be achieved by immersion in an ice bath, it is difficult to monitor and manage comatose or convulsing patients in an ice bath. Shivering may be provoked. Vigorous skin massage should follow immersion to prevent stasis.

(iii) Ice water soaks to body (especially the groin, neck and axilla areas). Good first aid measure. This, coupled with electric fan circulation of room air over the body, is a useful method in a medical centre without a BCU.

(iv) Ice water enemas and ice water gastric lavage. Less effective than skin cooling and may cause water intoxication.

7. Hypotension — volume resuscitate and start inotropes as indicated.

8. Disseminated Intravascular Coagulation (DIVC) — blood product support. Can consider low dose heparin.

9. Adjunctive measures: NG tube, urinary catheterisation, ECG monitoring, IV Chlorpropamazine 10–50 mg slowly q 6 hrs for vigorous shivering (may aggravate hypotension and interfere with sweating), IV diazepam is an alternative, treat convulsions with diazepam, peritoneal dialysis and cardiopulmonary bypass may be required for refractory cases (if adequate cooling not attainable after 1–2 hrs).

10. Antipyretics are NOT indicated.

11. Alcohol baths should not be used.

Prognosis

The intensity and duration of hyperpyrexia is inversely related to survival. Prompt cooling saves lives. Patients who remain in coma despite optimal management (> 8 hours) have a poor prognosis. Those that have a prolonged period of coma (> 3 hours) prior to regaining consciousness carry a higher risk of permanent sequelae (usually CNS). Patients with a transient period of coma (less than 3 hrs) usually make a complete recovery without any sequelae.

MEDICATIONS FOR TREATMENT OF COMMON SYMPTOMS

1. Commonly used medications for the management of nausea and vomiting — *Lim HL*

2. Giddiness and vertigo — *Ho HK*

3. Constipation — *Gwee KA*

4. Sedation — *Leong SO*

5. Wound care management — *Wong ST*

6. Medications for analgesia — *Lim HL*

COMMONLY USED MEDICATIONS FOR THE MANAGEMENT OF NAUSEA AND VOMITING

LIM HONG LIANG

Clinical evaluation

1. Always elucidate the cause of vomiting before giving symptomatic treatment.
2. Commonly encountered causes of nausea and vomiting in the wards:
   - (i) Gastroenteritis and food poisoning
   - (ii) Drug overdose
   - (iii) Drug-related: Cytotoxic chemotherapy, post-anaesthetic, opiates e.g. pethidine
   - (iv) Renal failure
   - (v) Vertigo and vestibular vomiting
   - (vi) Intestinal obstruction

Common available medications

Name (Trade name)	Preparation	Dosage	Remarks
Metoclopramide (Maxolon)	10 mg tab, 10 mg amp inj	10–20 mg 4–6x/d po/iv/im	Oculogyric crisis* Akathisia
Prochlorperazine (Stemetil)	5 mg tab 12.5 mg/amp inj	5–10 mg tds po 12.5 mg tds i/m	
Domperidome (Motilium)	10 mg tab	10–20 mg 3–4x/d po	
Ondansetron (Zofran)	8 mg tab 8 mg/amp inj 4 mg/amp inj	8 mg 1–3x/d po 8 mg 1–3x/d iv 24 mg/d CI	used in CINV** & PONV***
Granisetron (Kytril)	3 mg/amp inj 1 mg tab	3 mg/d iv (over 15 min)	used in CINV
Dexamethasone	0.5 mg/4 mg tab 4 mg/amp inj	see below under CINV	used in CINV
Lorazepam (Ativan)	0.5 mg/1 mg tab	1–2 mg 1–2x/d po	used in CINV

Name (Trade name)	Preparation	Dosage	Remarks
Haloperidol (Serenace)	0.5/1.5/5 mg tab 5 mg/amp inj	0.5 mg–2 mg 1–2x/d po/iv	used in CINV

* Management of oculogyric crisis/akathisia
  Benztropine (Cogentin)   1–2 mg iv
  Diazepam (valium)   5 mg slow iv   watch for respiratory depression
  Diphenhydramine (Benadryl) 25mg slow iv may cause sedation
** Chemotherapy induced nausea and vomiting
*** Post-operative nausea and vomiting

Management of Chemotherapy Induced Nausea and Vomiting

Nausea and vomiting is common for patients on cytotoxic chemotherapy. Severity depends on the emetic potential of the drug, dose administered, and the patient. However, with appropriate treatment, nausea and vomiting can be effectively prevented in the majority of cases. In most cases, the onset of nausea and vomiting occurs within hours of cytotoxic administration. But for cisplatin, the onset of chemotherapy may be delayed for more than 24–48 hours (delayed emesis), and can be severe and difficult to manage. For other patients, nausea and vomiting may occur before receiving the cytotoxics (anticipatory nausea and vomiting). This usually occurs in patients who had experienced bad nausea and vomiting during previous cycles of chemotherapy.

The emetic potential of cytotoxic agents can be classified as follows:

Severe	Moderate	Mild to None
Actinomycin D	Carboplatin	Bleomycin
Anthracyclines*	Cytarabine (<500mg/m^2)	Busulfan
Cisplatin	Cyclophosphamide (<600mg/m^2)	Chlorambucil
Cyclophosphamide (>600mg/m^2)	5-fluorouracil (>1g/m^2)	5-fluorouracil (<1g/m^2)

Severe	Moderate	Mild to None
Cytarabine ($>500mg/m^2$)	Hydroxyurea	Melphalan
Dacarbazine	L-asparaginase	Mercaptopurine
Ifosfamide	Methotrexate (>200 mg/m^2)	Methotrexate (<200 mg/m^2)
Mustine	Mitomycin Mitozantrone	Thiotepa Vinca alkaloids** Etoposide/Teniposide

*Anthracyclines   Includes daunorubicin, doxorubicin, epirubicin and idarubicin
**Vinca alkaloids Includes vincristine, vinorelbine, vinblastine and vindesine

Examples of antiemetic combinations

1. Highly emetogenic regimen — cisplatin containing regimen and high dose chemotherapy (in bone marrow transplant):
    (i)   ondansetron 8 mg iv immediately before and 8 mg iv bd, plus
    (ii)   oral metoclopramide 10–20 mg 6 hourly strictly, plus,
    (iii) oral dexamethasone 8 mg bd × 4 doses, followed by 4 mg bd x 4 doses, plus,
    (iv)   oral lorazepam 1 mg bd,
    (v)   granisetron iv 3 mg once daily (in 50 ml N/S over 15 min) can be used instead of ondansetron,
    (vi)   all anti-emetics to be given intravenously if vomiting occurs
    (vii) haloperidol may be added to the above if necessary.

2. Moderately emetogenic regimen — anthracycline containing regimen, usually given in outpatient:
    (i)   ondansetron 8 mg iv immediately before, plus
    (ii)   dexamethasone 8 mg iv immediately before, plus
    (iii) metoclopramide 10 mg po 6–8 hourly,
    (iv)   oral ondansetron 8 mg bd, dexamethasone 4 mg bd × 4 doses, lorazepam may be added if necessary.

3. Mildly emetogenic regimen — 5-fluorouracil, vincristine, oral melphalan, busulphan:
   (i)   metoclopramide 10 mg iv immediately before, plus
   (ii)   metoclopramide 10 mg po qds prn
   (iii) may be given without any anti-emetics.

GIDDINESS AND VERTIGO
HO KING HEE

Always elucidate the cause of vertigo/giddiness before symptomatic treatment. There are main categories of symptomatic treatment.

1. Labyrinthine sedatives — for symptomatic treatment of acute vertigo:
   (i)   Prochloperazine (Stemetil): IM 12.5 mg; oral 5 mg tds,
   (ii) Metoclopramide (Maxolon): IM or IV 10–20 mg; oral 10 mg tds,
   (iii) Cinnazarine (Sturgeron): Oral 25 mg tds.
   Administer parenterally for rapid effect or if patient cannot retain orally.
   Avoid chronic use because of risks of sedation, poor vestibular compensation, Parkinsonism, and psychological dependence.
   Acute use may result in oculogyric crisis — treat with IM benztropine 1–2 mg stat or IM or slow IV diphenhydramine 25 mg stat.

2. Non-specific agents — may relieve non-specific giddiness. Oral administration:
   (i)   Betahistidine 6–8 mg tds,
   (ii) Tanakan (gingko) 40 mg tds — qds,
   (iii) Duxaril 1 tab bd,
   (iv) Trimetazidine (Vasteral) 1 tab tds.

CONSTIPATION
GWEE KOK ANN

Constipation as a symptom: Reduced bowel frequency (normal ranges from 3 x/day to 3 x/week); hard or pellet stools, difficult passage requiring straining; feeling of incomplete evacuation.

Clinical evaluation
1. Define the patient's complaint. Is patient troubled by infrequent bowel movements, abdominal discomfort or painful defecation.
2. Determine if constipation is of recent onset (1–2 weeks) or longstanding (years).
3. In recent-onset constipation, suspect intestinal obstruction if any of the following is present: acute onset crampy abdominal pain, vomiting, abdominal tenderness or distension, absent or hyperactive bowel sounds, fluid levels on AXR. If intestinal obstruction suspected, rest the bowel, correct fluid and electrolytes intravenously and refer to the Surgical Service.
4. Look for treatable causes of constipation.

Causes of constipation
1. Functional, e.g. irritable bowel syndrome, idiopathic, depression, old age.
2. Drugs, e.g. narcotic analgesics, aluminum containing antacids, anticholinergics, tricyclic antidepressants.
3. Painful anal lesions, e.g. piles, fissures, solitary rectal ulcer.
4. Intestinal obstruction.
5. Metabolic or endocrine causes, e.g. dehydration, hypokalaemia, hypercalcaemia, hypothyroidism.
6. Neurological causes, e.g. post-operative ileus, CVA, diabetic neuropathy.

Common situations for laxative use or request

1. Elderly, immobile, debilitated or stroke patients: avoid mineral lubricants, e.g. Agarol because of increased risk of aspiration and decreased absorption of fat-soluble vitamins.
2. Angina, acute myocardial infarction, post-haemorrhoidectomy: stool softeners or lubricants preferred because they minimise straining at defecation.
3. Painful anal lesions: anti-inflamatory, anaesthetic ointments or suppositories preferred.
4. Hepatic encephalopathy: lactulose preferred, to produce 2 soft stools a day.

Cautions:

1. In renal failure or heart failure, avoid saline laxatives including Mg^{2+} and PO_4 containing oral and enema solutions.
2. Avoid laxatives in paralytic ileus.
3. Laxative use should be discouraged in the long-term management of constipation, which should involve adequate fluid and dietary fibre intake and life-style adjustments.

SEDATION
LEONG SEE ODD

Types of sedatives
1. Hypnotics.
2. Anxiolytics.
3. Barbiturates — seldom used as hypnotics because of risk of severe respiratory depression and dependence.

Indications
1. Insomnia — give oral agent at bedtime.
2. Anxiety disorders — give anxiolytic usually in divided doses throughout the day.
3. Acute confusional state or violent patient — parenteral route preferred.
4. Seizures — parenteral route to terminate episodes.
5. Premedication for procedures.

Prescribe sedatives cautiously in following conditions
1. Pulmonary insufficiency,
2. Liver disease,
3. Myasthenia gravis,
4. Patients already on medications that cause drowsiness, e.g. antihistamines, antipsychotics,
5. Pregnancy and breastfeeding.

Commonly used sedatives

Class	Common agents	Oral dose	Parenteral dose	Remarks
Benzodiazepine	Diazepam (Valium)	2–10 mg	IM/IV 5–10 mg	
	Lorazepam (Ativan)	1–2 mg	–	
	Midazolam (Dormicum)	7.5–15 mg	IM/IV 10–15 mg	
Cyclopyrrolone	Zopiclone (Imovane)	7.5–15 mg	–	
Chloral	Chloral hydrate	5–20 ml	–	Usually for children
Chlormethiazole	Chlormethiazole (heminevrin)	–	IV titrated to clinical status	Usually for status epilepticus
Paraldehyde	Paraldehyde	–	IM 5–10 ml	Relatively safe in pulmonary disease

WOUND CARE MANAGEMENT
WONG SOON TEE

Concept of ideal dressing
The ideal dressing keeps the wound moist but not macerated (moist wounds heal more rapidly than dry ones), at optimal conditions for healing and free from clinical infection and excessive slough.

Three phases of the wound healing process
1. Cleansing and removal of debris.
2. Granulation and vascularisation.
3. Epithelialisation.

Cleansing agents
1. Normal saline — for clean wounds, irrigate gently with copious quantities of normal saline to remove extraneous matter.
2. 0.05% chlorhexidine solution — antiseptic of choice for heavily colonised wounds; mildly toxic to granulation tissue.
3. 6% hydrogen peroxide — reserve for very dirty wounds; do not use for >1 week because toxic to granulation tissue.

Debriding agents
1. Surgical debridement — should be employed early if patient's general condition allows it.
2. Chemical debridement with proteolytic enzymes (e.g. Varidase, Elase) — discontinue once devitalised tissue removed because damages healthy tissue.
3. Autolytic debridement with hydrocolloid dressings (e.g. Duoderm, Comfeel) — slower than surgical method, cannot be used if clinical infection present.
4. Mechanical debridement using wet-to-dry gauze dressing (painful, non-selectively removes both healthy and necrotic tissue); by irrigation.

Selection of wound-care materials

1. Black and necrotic wounds — Surgical debridement of choice; otherwise proteolytic enzyme or hydrocolloid dressing.
2. Yellow and sloughy wounds — as in (1) above; followed by hydrogel dressings, e.g. Intrasite gel, Duoderm hydrogel.
3. Granulating tissue — either paraffin gauze, calcium alginate dressing (e.g. Algoderm, Kaltostat), hydrocolloid dressing or hydrogel dressing.
4. Epithelialising wound — hydrocolloid dressing.
5. Infected wounds are recognised by pain, increase in discharge or slough, erythema and induration at the edges and/or cellulitis. Systemic antibiotics indicated. Treat wound with normal saline irrigation or chlorhexidine packing, then calcium alginate or hydrogel dressings.

Topical antibiotics

Role not established. If used, prescribe only for limited duration to avoid colonisation with resistant organisms:

1. Silver sulphadiazine — both Gram positive and negative organisms,
2. Mupirocin (Bactroban) — effective against Staphylococci including MRSA, Streptococci.
3. Bacitracin — effective against Gram positive organisms.

MEDICATIONS FOR ANALGESIA
LIM HONG LIANG

Clinical evaluation

1. Always elucidate the cause of pain before giving symptomatic treatment. If an acute abdomen is suspected, do not give analgesics till a diagnosis is reached. In case of doubt, consult a more senior doctor.

2. For most forms of pain, it is appropriate to start with simple, non-opiate oral analgesics, reserving opiates for severe or terminal cancer pain.

3. Avoid use of NSAIDs in patients with peptic ulcer disease or dyspepsia, renal impairment, and in cardiac failure.

4. When using opiates:

    (i) Constipation is a common side effect. Prophylax with senokot 2 tabs on, increase to 2 tabs bd if required. Lactulose prn/regular dosing may be required in some.

    (ii) Nausea may be experienced by about one third of patients when treatment with opiates is initiated. However, tolerance develops early, usually in 5–7 days, and nausea usually subsides quickly. Symptomatic treatment with maxolon or stemetil is effective in most.

    (iii) Other side effects include excessive sedation, respiratory depression, CNS effects (confusion, hallucination, nightmare), urinary retention, pruritus and hypotension.

    (iv) Use with care in the following groups of patients

Renal impairment	action increased and prolonged
Liver impairment	may precipitate hepatic encephalopathy
Respiratory conditions	cause respiratory depression, especially in COAD patients
Urinary outlet obstruction	may precipitate acute urinary retention
Hypotensive patients	worsens blood pressure

| Head injury | masks CNS signs |
| Acute abdomen | masks serious intra-abdominal pathology |

Common preparations available for pain-relief

Name (trade name)	Preparation	Dosage	Remarks
Paracetamol	500 mg tab soluble tabs syrup	0.5–1 g 3–4x/d po	maximum 4g/d liver toxicity, esp if >8g/d
Non-steriodal anti-inflammatory drugs (NSAIDS)			
Aspirin	300 mg tab enteric coated tab 100 mg	300–650 mg 3–4x/d 650–1300 mg 3–4x/d	analgesic dose anti-inflammatory dose
Diclofenac sodium (Voltaren/Voltaren SR)	25 mg/50 mg tab 100 mg SR tb 12.5/50 mg supp	75–250 mg/d in 2–3 doses SR tab – once daily	
	75 mg/amp inj	75 mg im	IM for initial therapy only
Ibuprofen	200/400 mg tab	200–400 mg 2–4x/d	max 2.4 g/d
Indomethacin (Indocid)	25 mg cap 50 mg supp	25–50 mg tds supp on or bd	max 200 mg/d
Ketoprofen (Oruvail)	100/200 mg cap SR	100–200 mg om	
Mefenamic acid (Ponstan)	250/mg cap	250–500 mg tds	
Naproxen sodium (Synflex)	275/550 mg tab	550–100 mg/d in 2–3 divided doses	
Piroxicam (Brexine)	10/20 mg cap	10–20 mg daily in 1–2 divided doses	
Sulindac (Clinoril)	150 mg tab	150 mg bd	
Opiates			
Codeine	30 mg tab	30–60 mg tds	
Tramadol (Tramal)	50 mg cap 50 mg/amp inj	50–100 mg 3–4x/d inj: SC/IM/IV	max 400 mg/d
Buprenorphine (Temgesic)	0.2 mg tab S/L	0.2–0.4 tabs S/L 6–8 hrly	
	0.3 mg/amp inj	0.3–0.6 mg IM 6–8 hrly	
Pentazocine (Talwin)	25 mg tab 30 mg/amp inj	25–50 mg 4 hrly 30 mg 3–4 hrly SC/IM/IV	max: 360 mg/d

Name (trade name)	Preparation	Dosage	Remarks
Pethidine	50 mg/100 mg/amp inj	1 mg/kg 4–6 hrly IM	IV bolus hazardous
Morphine	10 mg/amp inj	0.1–0.15 mg/kg 4 hrly SC/IM Continuous infusion 0.5–2 mg/h	IV bolus hazardous
	1 mg/ml syrup	5–40 mg po 4 hrly	Lower starting dose in elderly
(MST Continous)	30 mg tab SR	bd dosing	see below for dosing
Fentanyl	Transdermal patch 25 ug/hr, 50 ug/h 100 ug/h	change every 72 hours	may cause fatal respiratory depression see below for dosing
Combination Panadeine	paracetamol 500 mg codeine 8 mg	1–2 tabs 6–8 hrly	
Beserol	paracetamol 450 mg chlormezanone 100 mg	1–2 tabs 6–8 hrly	

GUIDELINES FOR TREATMENT OF CANCER PAIN

LIM HONG LIANG

Selection of Appropriate Agent

Mild pain	Non-opiates analgesics (Step 1)	Paracetamol NSAIDs
Moderate pain	Step 2 opiates	Tramadol Codeine Panadeine +/– non-opiod treatment
Severe pain	Step 3 opiates	morphine fentanyl patch +/– non-opiod treatment

Adjuvant therapy

Pharmacologic agents	Steroids	– general well being, and pain relief in nerve compression, increased intracranial pressure, etc
	Antidepressants	– neuropathic pain, improve underlying depression, and insomnia
	Anticonvulsants	– neuropathic pain
	Diphosphonates	– painful bony metastases
Radiation	Radiotherapy	– relief of pain due to local tumour involvement
	strontium	– for pain due to widespread metastatic bony metastases
Neural blockage	e.g. coeliac plexus neurolysis, chemical sympathectomy, intrathecal neurolysis	
Others	Heat treatment, relaxation, etc.	

Dosing of analgesics

1. Titrate the dose of each agent against patient's pain until pain is adequately relieved, or until maximum dose is reached.
2. Prescribe analgesics regularly and not prn for persistent pain.
3. Use optimal dose interval, e.g. mist morphine should be given 4 hourly and not 6 or 8 hourly.
4. PRN dosing should be used for breakthrough pain in addition to (not instead of) regular administration of analgesics.
5. Use oral route whenever possible.

GENERAL PRESCRIBING INFORMATION FOR OPIOD ANALGESICS

Approximate equivalent analgesics dosing when converting oral to parental or vice versa

	Parental	Oral
Morphine	10 mg	30 mg
Codeine	130 mg	200 mg

Approximate equivalent analgesic dosing when converting one preparation to another

Tramadol 50 mg = Codeine 60 mg = codeine 30 mg + acetaminophen 650 mg

Fentanyl patch	Oral morphine
25 ug/hr	45–134 mg/day
50 ug/hr	135–224 mg/day
75 ug/hr	225–314 mg/day
100 ug/hr	315–404 mg/day

When switching from one opiod to another, in patients whose pain is well controlled, the initial dose of the new opiod should be 25% to 50% less than the equivalent dose to allow for incomplete cross tolerance.

Fentanyl Patch
Fatal respiratory depression can occur
Do not use in patients naive to opoids

Morphine Syrup
1. Comes in a concentration of 1 mg/ml.
2. Morphine preparation of choice for patient starting on step 3 opiates.
3. Starting dose is 5 ml 4 hourly.
4. Increase by 5 ml 4 hourly every 1 to 2 days until adequate pain control is achieved.
5. Dosing may be reduced in elderly patients, or in patients with respiratory disorders.

Controlled Release Morphine
MST Continus – controlled release preparation
30 mg strength tablets
1. Patient should not be started on controlled release morphine for initial pain control.
2. Dose should be worked out from the total daily dose of mist morphine for optimal pain control.
3. For example, if the patient require mist morphine 10 ml 4 hourly, the daily dose will be 60 mg/day
4. Once the pain control is stable, this can be converted to MST Continus 30 mg bd (total 60 mg/day)
5. Controlled release morphine is preferred for chronic pain control as bd dosing interval is convenient.
6. Main disadvantage is cost.

Continuous Morphine Infusion
This can be given as iv infusion, as used in post-operative pain control or for acute pain control in the intensive care unit. In chronic cancer pain control, parental morphine, when required, is usually given via the s/c route. In the Department of Medical Oncology, s/c morphine infusion is

usually administered using the Deltec ambulatory pump, a walkman sized pump that can be carried easily.

Again, the total daily dose of s/c morphine required can be worked up by dividing the amount of daily oral morphine dose by 3, or if patient was on intermittent s/c morphine injection prior to switching to s/c infusion, the dose can be obtained by adding the number of doses required in a 24 hour period.

Patient Controlled Analgesia (PCA)

In Deltec pumps designed specifically for morphine administration, in addition to delivering a constant background dose of morphine, additional intermittent boluses can be delivered by pressing a button on the pump. Size of the boluses can be pre-programmed, with ranges from 1 to more than 10 mg depending on the need, and the minimal time interval in between 2 boluses can also be pre-determined, in order to safeguard against overdosage. In this way, the patient can control the amount of morphine for optimal pain control. The background dose of morphine infusion can then be adjusted according to the number of additional boluses required in the previous 24 hours. Again, the pump is available in the Department of Medical Oncology.

Request for use of the Deltac pump can be channelled through the Medical Oncology Registrar on call.